Early Years Practitioner:
a Level 2 Textbook

For Baillière Tindall:

Senior Commissioning Editor: Ninette Premdas
Project Development Manager: Karen Gilmour
Project Manager: Jane Dingwall
Designer Direction: George Ajayi

Early Years Practitioner: a Level 2 Textbook

FOURTH EDITION

Maureen O'Hagan BEd MSc MIHE RGN NNEB

Director of Quality Assurance,
Council for Awards in Children's Care and Education,
St Albans, Hertfordshire;
President of the National Association of Nursery Nurses;
UK Secretary of OMEP

Baillière Tindall

EDINBURGH LONDON NEW YORK PHILADELPHIA ST LOUIS SYDNEY TORONTO 2001

BAILLIÈRE TINDALL
An imprint of Harcourt Publishers Limited

© Baillière Tindall 1997
© Harcourt Publishers Limited 2001

 is a registered trademark of Harcourt Publishers Limited

First published 1981
Second edition 1988
Third edition 1997
Fourth edition 2001

0 7020 2608 5

British Library Cataloguing in Publication Data
A catalogue record for this book is available from the British Library

Library of Congress Cataloging in Publication Data
A catalog record for this book is available from the Library of Congress

Note
Medical knowledge is constantly changing. As new information
becomes available, changes in treatment, procedures, equipment and
the use of drugs become necessary. The author and the publishers have
taken care to ensure that the information given in this text is accurate
and up to date. However, readers are strongly advised to confirm that
the information, especially with regard to drug usage, complies with
the latest legislation and standards of practice.

The
publisher's
policy is to use
**paper manufactured
from sustainable forests**

Printed in China

Contents

Preface

I started writing this book as a fourth edition of *Geraghty's Caring for Children*. However, there have been so many changes in training, such as the latest version of National Occupational Standards, vocational qualifications for early years care and education and also in recent child care initiatives that the publishers agreed that as this was really a totally new book a change of title would be appropriate.

In recent years a large number of very important changes have been and are still taking place in the field of early years care and education. The Qualifications and Curriculum Authority (QCA) has produced a framework of qualifications for those working in childcare and education and playwork*. In order for qualifications to gain a place on the framework they have to be written in accordance with QCA requirements. The framework has three vertical columns: column 1 has the job roles; column 2 has the vocational qualifications; and column 3 has the National Vocational Qualifications (NVQs). There are also horizontal lines, which divide the qualifications and job roles into levels 2 and 3. This book is aimed at those people who are undertaking a level 2 qualification.

The present Government has introduced a number of initiatives within the National Childcare Strategy which are intended to increase the number of child care places available to parents and enhance existing provision. This has led to very active recruitment drives for staff at all levels and in all types of early years care and education work. It has also led to new types of funding for training and the Early Years Development Partnerships are one of the new key players to be given funding to enable them to train new and existing staff.

---

* The latest information on the QCA framework can be seen at the QCA website: www.qca.org.uk

This book is a tool for those in training to gain underpinning knowledge and understanding about children and their families. It is predominantly written for those studying at level 2 but there is an overlap of topics, which could also help those who are studying at level 3. Each chapter has a signpost at the beginning, which links the reader with the relevant vocational qualification modules and NVQ units. Chapters have scenarios throughout and the answers to these can be put into a candidate's portfolio as evidence for underpinning knowledge. At the end of each chapter there are assignments and practical activities which can be used as underpinning knowledge evidence. The practical activities can be undertaken in the candidate's workplace or placement.

I have tried to make the book as user friendly as possible whilst using a form of language that will suit all age groups. I am very aware that a large number of candidates are women returners who are coming into child care as a new career for themselves.

At the time of writing all information in the book is correct, however, new research may rapidly change the way we deal with certain situations. Therefore, before giving information to parents on matters such as meningitis, cot deaths, salt intake for young children, etc. it is as well to check with the head of your establishment or the relevant national organisation (addresses at the end of the book). I hope that you enjoy reading the book and will learn a great deal and I wish you luck in your assessment and future career.

London 2001   Maureen O'Hagan

ACKNOWLEDGEMENTS To Mike, Rodan and other family and friends for their tolerance of my neglect of them whilst I have been writing.

DISCLAIMER Please note that the views expressed in this book are those of the author and are not necessarily the views of her employer.

PUBLISHER'S ACKNOWLEDGEMENTS All photographs, except those on pages 123, 128, 171 and 205, were provided by Joss Reiver Bany © 1997 and feature the children, staff and parents of Lea View Community Nursery, Springfield, London E5: our grateful thanks to all involved. The photographs on pages 123 and 128, of Nathaniel and Bethany James, were provided by Sarah James.

Chapter 1

Working with Children

This chapter links with the following unit for the National Vocational Qualifications (NVQs) in Early Years Care and Education: the underlying principles which underpin good practice. This chapter also links with CACHE Diploma units, particularly Unit 10 and Certificate Unit 4.

INTRODUCTION

All those wishing to work with children need to have knowledge and understanding of the child's wider role as a member of a family. There is a need to understand the different patterns of families and how these work as social units. Historically, the role of the child within society has moved from the child being treated as a mini-adult with no feelings (15th–16th century) through to the late 20th century where the needs of the child are paramount. Such changes reflect the way that society has changed and evolved.

Child care workers[1] also need to work in partnership with parents or the child's primary care-giver in order to ensure that all the child's needs are met. This requires the child care worker to have an understanding of family life and the factors which mitigate against families such as poverty, unemployment, racism, prejudice etc. Child care workers need to help build the parents' confidence by ensuring that they know that the child is safe in their care. In order to promote good practice, child care workers need to be understanding of children and adults, non-judgmental and committed to offering high quality child care and education. There is at present no official 'Code of Practice' for child care workers but the National Occupational Standards for Early Years Care and Education has the following set of underlying principles which underpin good practice when working with children and their families:

■ The welfare of the child
   The welfare of the child is paramount. All early years workers must give precedence to the rights and well being of the children they work with. Children should be listened to and their opinions

[1] Throughout the text people working with children will be referred to as 'child care workers'; however this is purely for ease in reading as the correct title should be 'child care and education workers', education and care being indivisible in the role.

and concerns treated seriously. Management of children's behaviour should emphasize positive expectations for that behaviour, and responses to unwanted behaviour should be suited to the child's stage in development. A child must never be slapped, smacked or humiliated.

- Working in partnership with parents/families
  Parents and families occupy a central position in their children's lives, and early years workers must respect that role. Parents and families should be listened to as experts on their own children. Information about children's development and progress should be shared openly with parents. Respect must be shown for families' traditions and child care practices, and every effort made to comply with parents' wishes for their children.

- Children's learning and development
  Children learn more rapidly in their earliest years than at any other time in life. Development and learning in these earliest years lay the foundations for abilities, characteristics and skills later in life. Learning begins at birth. The care and education of children are interwoven.

  Children should be offered a range of experiences and activities which support all aspects of their development – social, physical, intellectual, communication and emotional. The choice of experiences and activities (the 'curriculum') should depend on accurate assessment of the stage of development reached by a child, following observation and discussion with families. Early years workers have varying responsibilities concerning the planning and implementation of the curriculum, according to their work role, but all contributions to such planning and implementation should set high expectations for children and build on their achievements and interests. Child-initiated play activities should be recognized and valued, as well as the adult planned curriculum. Written records should be kept of children's progress, and these records should be shared with parents.

- Equality of opportunity
  All children should be offered equality of access to opportunities to learn and develop, and so work towards their potential. Each child is a unique individual; early years workers must respect this individuality; children should not be treated 'all the same'. In order to meet a child's needs, it is necessary to treat each child 'with equal concern'; some children need more and/or different support in order to have equality of opportunity. It is essential to avoid stereotyping children on the basis of gender, racial origins,

cultural or social background (including religion, language, class and family pattern), or disability; such stereotypes may act as barriers to equality of access to opportunity. Early years workers should demonstrate their valuing of children's racial and other personal characteristics in order to help them develop self-esteem.

■ Anti-discrimination

Early years workers must not discriminate against any child, family or group in society on the grounds of gender, racial origins, cultural or social background (including religion, language, class and family pattern), disability or sexuality. They must acknowledge and address any personal beliefs or opinions which prevent them respecting the value systems of other people, and comply with legislation and the policies of their work setting relating to discrimination. Children learn prejudice from the earliest years and must be provided with accurate information to help them avoid prejudice. Expressions of prejudice by children or adults should be challenged, and support offered to those children or adults who are the objects of prejudice and discrimination. Early years workers have a powerful role to play in nurturing greater harmony amongst various groups in our society for future generations.

■ Confidentiality

Information about children and families must never be shared with others, without the permission of the family, except in the interests of protecting children. Early years workers must adhere to the policy of their work setting concerning confidential information, including passing information to colleagues. Confidentiality must also be maintained with information about other workers.

■ Keeping children safe

Work practices should help to prevent accidents to children and adults and protect their health. Emergency procedures of the work setting, including record keeping, must be adhered to. All early years workers have a responsibility to contribute to the protection of children from abuse, according to their work role.

■ Celebrating diversity

Britain is a multi-racial, multi-cultural society. The contributions made to this society by a variety of cultural groups should be viewed in a positive light, and information about varying traditions, customs and festivals should be presented to children as a source of pleasure and enjoyment. Children should be helped to develop a sense of their identity within their racial, cultural and social groups, as well as having the opportunity to learn about cultures different from their own. No one culture should be represented as superior to any other; pride in one's own cultural and social background does not require condemnation of that of other people.

- Working with other professionals
  Advice and support should be sought from other professionals in the best interests of the children and families, and information shared with them, subject to the principle of confidentiality. Respect should be shown for the roles of other professionals.
- The reflective practitioner
  Early years workers should use any opportunity they are offered or which arises to reflect on their practice and principles, and make use of the conclusions from such reflection in developing and extending practice. Seeking advice and support to help resolve queries or problems should be seen as a form of strength and professionalism. Opportunities for in-service training and continuous professional development should be used to the maximum.

Whilst these underlying principles may appear to be complex, they do form the basis of good practice. A number of the concepts in the underlying principles are explored in the chapters of this book.

Present day society in the UK is culturally pluralistic; this means that it is made up of people from many cultures and religions. For the child care worker the most important point when dealing with children is that there is a duty to ensure that all the needs of each child are met, regardless of that child's age, gender, ethnicity, religion or ability/disability. Anti-bias practice is the basis of all good child care practice. This chapter will examine different family structures, factors which mitigate against families and the anti-discriminatory/anti-bias practices which all child care and education workers need to incorporate into their own practice.

DIFFERENT TYPES OF FAMILY

Respect for families requires understanding of the composition of the family. Most children live in a family unit but there are a number of different types of family unit of which the child care worker needs to be aware.

The family unit is a microcosm of the wider society; in other words it is a mini-reflection of the wider society. When a child lives with a family it will be introduced by the family to the values and norms of the wider society. Children will believe that the way things are done in their family is the way all families do things. It is only when they get older and visit other children's homes or exchange experiences with other children that they may realize that there are differences between families. It is important that child care workers do not undermine a child's family for however disorganized it may appear to the adult it is a very crucial part of a child's life.

The Extended Family

The *Collins Dictionary of Sociology* defines the extended family as:

> A group of people, related by kinship, where more than two generations of relatives live together (or in close proximity), usually forming a single household.

The most famous study of extended families in the UK was carried out by Young & Wilmott (1962) when they looked at family life in Bethnal Green in East London during the 1950s. If you read this book it will give you some idea of how extended families in Britain operated. However, due to changes in housing and people moving around the country in order to find work, there are very few extended families of the Young and Wilmott type left in the UK.

In order to study the extended family in present times it is necessary to look beyond Europe and the Western world to countries such as Asia, Africa and South America.

Children born into the extended family will have the advantage of being able to bond with a number of adults who are all likely to take a part in the child rearing process. Studies have shown that within the extended family it is the women who have the strongest networks, helping each other with tasks such as child care, cooking, shopping, doing the laundry and other domestic tasks. Much of the decision making is undertaken by the whole family and is based upon what is best for the family as a whole, not necessarily on what is best for the individual. (However, within some religions, for example Islam, the final decision may be left to the eldest male in the family and this may cause problems if the male concerned is in a different country from the members of the family he is making decisions about.)

Extended families protect their members, and if there is a crisis it is most likely that family members will be consulted before help is sought from outside agencies. It is a close knit situation which offers advantages and disadvantages to its members.

Many people have found strength in being a member of an extended family as they are able to have support and help whenever they need it. Children are cared for within the broader family network, and it offers care and support to all its members. It is particularly useful for new parents and the elderly.

However, some people have found this type of family situation too suffocating as it inhibits individuality and privacy. Extended families place great pressure upon their members to conform to the family norms and values, and this can lead to conflict situations.

The Nuclear Family

The nuclear family is a small unit consisting of two adults and their children. It is the commonest form of family unit now found in the UK and Europe. With high divorce rates it is also very common to find that one of the adults may be a step-parent. Burgoyne & Clark (1982) estimated that in the UK, 7% of all children under the age of 17 years live with a step-parent. It is also quite common to find a couple living together with their children without being married.

Within an industrial society the nuclear family is the most economical type of living unit. It requires small living accommodation and offers independence from parents and other family members. It enables the family to move around the country easily in order to follow their work.

Within the nuclear family the adults are able to decide which of the wider family relations they will keep contact with and how frequently they will meet as a wider family. Nuclear families restrict the number of adults who are available for the child to relate to and in many instances prevent aunts, uncles and grandparents from taking a role in the child rearing process. Whilst the nuclear family is able to offer advantages in our present day society, it has also been blamed by politicians and others for a lot of the problems which have arisen in families, such as the high incidence of divorce, family violence and child abuse. Many nuclear families do not have the support of relatives close by who can help out in times of need; this puts an added stress upon the adults in the family who may be struggling to cope.

Lone Parent Families

According to Moss (1988), one in 10 households with a child under 10 years of age were lone parent families. A family may only have one parent due to death of one of the parents, separation, divorce or a woman producing a child outside of a relationship. Moss (1988), in his study of families in the 12 member states of the European Economic Union, found that the UK had the highest figures for divorce. This in turn led to a large number of lone parent families in the UK. Families where one of the parents is serving a prison sentence or may be a soldier on active service experience the same problems as other lone parent families.

Lone parents often find themselves in isolated positions with little or no support from members of their immediate family, who may live too far away to be of any assistance on a daily basis. Many lone parent families have to rely on income support, as they are unable to work if they have small children. If they do manage to find part-time employment it is usually poorly paid and does not always cover the high costs that they may have to pay for child care. It must be remembered that not all lone parent families are 'problem families' and therefore do not qualify for a place for their child in a day nursery, family centre or other local authority supported provision. One of the greatest problems for lone parent families is trying to bring up a family on a low income; many families struggle to keep poverty at bay. Not all lone parent families are poor as a number of career women consciously choose to have a child and not to live with the father. These women may earn very good salaries that enable them to support their children without needing help from state benefits.

Reconstituted Families

This is the term that is used to describe the situation when two divorced people marry and form a family unit. With the very high divorce rate in the UK (it is the highest in Europe), this type of family is a very common social unit. Two previously married people coming together may result in them both becoming step-parents to children from the previous marriages. It may bring two groups of children into one family and there may also be children from the second marriage.

In many cases this type of family can work very well, but in some cases there may be resentment, rivalry and rancour that lead to stress and tension within the family. Being a step-parent is not an easy task and can be particularly difficult if the step-parents have children of their own. They will need to make a conscious effort not to put their own children's needs before the needs of the step-children. Step-parents have not in the past had good images in children's stories where they are often depicted as nasty, ugly and cruel (you only have to think of Cinderella). Many traditional stories have based their plots upon the theme of the wicked step-parent (usually step-mother). From such stories young children may have a very distorted view of what step-parents are like and this may cause them fear and distress. Children may also be resentful of the person who has displaced their real mother or father, whom they are now only able to see at weekends and holidays. Step-parents have to make very conscious efforts in order to build up relationships with their step-children. Step-parenting requires a great deal of sensitivity and understanding, and an acknowledgement from these parents that on many occasions they will find themselves in a 'no win' situation.

SCENARIO 1.1

Melanie, aged 4 years, lives with her father and new stepmother Sarah. Recently Melanie has begun to exhibit behaviour problems at the nursery. She has temper tantrums, is always demanding attention from the staff and if she is not given it she becomes aggressive. On talking to Sarah you find that Melanie is behaving in the same way at home. Explain what you think is causing Melanie's change in behaviour and describe what the nursery can do to help Melanie.

FACTORS WHICH MITIGATE AGAINST FAMILIES

Social Class and Home Life

The influence of the home upon the child has long lasting effects. It is the major influence upon the child during its first years of life. The effects of social class upon child rearing practices were clearly illustrated in a number of research projects carried out by John and Elizabeth Newsom in the late 1960s/1970s (Newsom & Newsom 1976). More recently, Barbara Tizard et al (1988) in *Young Children at School in the Inner City* examined, amongst other things, the class factor and its relationship to those children who were underachievers.

The value system of the home will determine the way the family will rear its children. For example, the aristocracy use nannies as a preparation for the child going away to public school, whereas the middle classes may use nannies in order to enable the mother to continue her career. Research has shown that the middle classes make maximum use of pre-school facilities, whilst the working classes may feel that preparation for education is a waste of time as it has done nothing to help them in their search for a better lifestyle. However, it is significant that research has also shown that densely populated inner city working class areas are often poorly serviced with pre-school facilities, so working class parents who do value pre-school education may not have the facilities available to their children.

The home determines the language that the child will speak and the value system that the child will be introduced to. Basil Bernstein undertook considerable research in this area and put forward the theory that there are two language codes: the elaborated code, which is not context bound and is easily understood by all; and the restricted code, which is context bound and therefore difficult to understand outside the context to which it refers. Bernstein associated these codes with class stratification but other researchers have found that all people operate between the two codes. In some cases a child's home language may not be English and many under-fives are very successfully bilingual, moving easily between the language of the home and the language of the wider society.

The family will determine which toys children are given to play with, where they are taken on outings, whom they play with or are friends with etc. The family will also decide whether activities are undertaken as a family group, on an individual basis or whether older siblings are responsible for organizing the activities for the younger members of the family. Parental expectations also have a significant effect upon children's development. Such expectations range from the way children behave in different situations to what clothes they will be expected to wear, what activities they will participate in and how they progress through the education system.

The economic circumstances of the family will often have a bearing on the type of activities that a child may participate in. If the family has a car and money to spare, then outings will often happen on a regular basis and be away from the immediate home environment. Using public transport with small children can be a very daunting task, particularly for lone parents, and in these families activities are likely to take place closer to home.

Poverty

Poverty can affect families from all different social classes. We live in a society, which is consumer orientated, but one is only able to consume if the money is available. Oppenheim (1993) points out that '... poverty is about social exclusion imposed by an inadequate income. It is not only about having to go short of food or clothing, it is also about not being able to join a local sports club, or send your children on a school trip, or go out with friends or have a Christmas dinner.' Kumar (1993) states that in 1991 nearly one in every three children in the country was living in poverty. Not all poverty is due to unemployment: in a large number of cases, parents have employment but they earn far below the national average; others are sick or have disabilities, which prevent them from working. However, unemployment has been a major cause of poverty amongst the middle classes who had what they thought were secure jobs for life within professions such as banking, accountancy, marketing etc. Many of these people have had their homes repossessed by mortgage companies and have had to undergo a very drastic change in lifestyle. As the unemployment figures rise, so do the numbers of children who find themselves in poor households. Nina Oldfield in 1991 found that the weekly cost of a child was on average:

£56.50 for a child aged 4 or 10 and £57.82 for a child aged 10 or 16 assuming that his/her parents are local authority tenants. £58.54 for a child aged 4 or 10 and £59.72 for a child aged 10 or 16 living in owner-occupied accommodation. (Quoted in Oppenheim 1993, p. 62)

There are government benefits for those people who are low paid, such as the Working Families Tax Credit (which gives money to generate a minimum income of up to £200 per week to families with children with at least one full time earner) and Childcare Tax Credits (which are able to help low earners with their charges for child care up to a limit of £100 for a family with one child). These benefits are intended to bring the low income up to the poverty line. The present government has taken social exclusion seriously and in its Annual Report (HMSO 1999) 'Opportunity for All: tackling poverty and social exclusion' it sets out the new initiatives which it has implemented; these include the National Childcare Strategy, the Sure Start Programme, Literacy and Numeracy Projects, Education Action Zones and Working Family Tax Credits.

The effects that poverty has upon families are many, not least being the loss of self-esteem and worth as useful members of society, and a poor quality of life. Bradshaw (1990) offers the following list of the impact and long term consequences of poverty on children:

- Physical which include
  - Infant mortality
  - Childhood deaths
  - Child morbidity
  - Child development
    Height
    Weight
    Nutrition
  - Racial disadvantage
  - Homelessness and housing conditions
  - Clothing
  - Child protection
  - Child abuse
- Behavioural which include
  - Education
  - Truancy
  - Teenage conceptions
  - Pocket money

- Child labour
- TV viewing
- Smoking
- Drinking
- Drugs
- Juvenile crime.

Obviously a number of the effects on Bradshaw's list will not affect small children directly, but could certainly have an effect upon the family as a whole. It also needs to be remembered that unemployment rates for black and ethnic minority people have always been higher than the unemployment rates for white people (Oppenheim 1993), and even if they have qualifications, these people are still more likely to have difficulty in finding employment. There are more women than men who are in low-paid employment, particularly as low pay is associated with part-time employment. There has been marginal improvement in the rates of pay for low paid workers since the government signed up to the European Directive on a minimum national wage, which it set at £3.60 per hour for people over 18 years of age and £3.00 per hour for those 18 years old and under. However, some critics have stated that this has led to greater unemployment and fewer employment opportunities when the employer is either too small an organization to be able to afford to pay the minimum wage e.g. a playgroup, or where the employer has cut back on staff numbers in order to save the extra salary costs.

The child care worker needs to be aware of these facts and of the necessity to treat those from poor families with respect and understanding. Child care workers can ensure that children from these families are encouraged in order to build up their self-esteem and confidence so that they benefit as much as possible from attending a playgroup, nursery or school.

Homelessness

It has already been mentioned above that the loss of employment could also result in a family becoming homeless. In the 1980s there was a lot of government encouragement for people to buy their own homes, including those people living in local authority accommodation. Following this boom, the UK experienced a recession and many people lost their jobs as companies folded or cut back on the numbers of workers they were employing. People with mortgages found that they were unable to pay them, and the mortgage companies repossessed their homes, leaving families homeless. When a family with young children becomes homeless the local authority has a duty to find the mother and the children accommodation. For many families the first stage is to be placed in temporary accommodation, which may be bed-and-breakfast accommodation. In 1990 the London Boroughs Association estimated that there were 9000 or more children living in bed-and-breakfast accommodation in London (Kumar 1993). Families were likely to stay in bed-and-breakfast for anything from 50–67 weeks whilst waiting for the local authority to find them a permanent home. Very few local authorities are able to offer council owned accommodation and they liaise with housing associations in order to provide housing for those in need. As previously mentioned, the local authority only has a duty to provide accommodation for the mother and children; the father will have to find himself accommodation elsewhere. This effectively splits up the family and may lead to a permanent family breakdown. Living in temporary accommodation can have serious effects upon the physical, emotional and mental health of all the family members.

A second option for families who may have lost their home is to move in with relatives. Whilst this may seem preferable to living in bed-and-breakfast accommodation, it can lead to overcrowding, quarrels and stresses for the resident family and the incomers. There are no accurate figures for the numbers of families living in this situation, as they may not come to the attention of the local authority or social services. Lack of amenities and lack of privacy can lead to marital conflict and maternal depression. Child care workers need to remember that children living in temporary accommodation, in cramped conditions or in high rise flats will need extra opportunities for boisterous physical play which will develop their large muscle coordination and help them release excess energy.

Family Violence

As families find themselves in stressful situations and unable to cope with their problems there is a greater likelihood of family violence. Resorting to alcohol or drugs to 'drown their sorrows' can lead to normally tolerant people becoming violent. There are many reasons why violence may occur in families, such as low tolerance levels, lack of parenting skills, and/or pressures from outside the family such as poverty, unemployment, poor housing etc. Children of such families are more often the victims of violence than the perpetrators.

Although children may live in a household where there is violence between the parents or other adults, violence might not be shown towards the children. However, research undertaken by the NSPCC has shown a correlation between child abuse and domestic violence: in 45% of child abuse cases the mother was also being abused (Calouste Gulbenkian 1995). Violence may not just be physical, as the Women's Aid Federation of England (Calouste Gulbenkian 1995) states:

> Violence can also mean among other things: threats, deprivation of food, limiting contact with family or friends, constant criticism, being locked in the house, intimidation, threatening children to exert power and control over women, stealing money from women or depriving them of money.

Children living in these situations are caught in a conflict between both parents; this in turn causes stress-related illnesses, emotional confusion, acceptance of abuse as a 'norm' of family life, guilt, isolation, fear and the likelihood that they will become abusing adults. Child care workers need to be sensitive in their handling of these children and help them regain their self-esteem and confidence. It is important that the adults in child care and education establishments encourage a non-violent atmosphere by promoting cooperative games, negotiating skills, sharing activities and teaching children how they can help each other. Discouraging aggressive games with guns and other weapons and stories about violence, and dealing promptly with children who bully or threaten others will also make the children feel that there is a safe, secure, non-violent atmosphere in the nursery.

SCENARIO 1.2

Vicki is 3 years old and attends your playgroup for five morning sessions a week. You are aware that Vicki and her mother and older brother are living in bed-and-breakfast accommodation. Write a list of what you think will be Vicki's needs, which arise from her home situation. Draw up a programme of activities for Vicki and explain how these will answer her particular needs.

PROMOTING ANTI-DISCRIMINATORY/ ANTI-BIAS PRACTICE

One of the fundamental principles of the Children Act 1989 is that the welfare of the child is paramount and that all children's needs must be met regardless of the child's age, sex, religion, race or ability. In order for carers to meet these needs they must have knowledge and understanding of the principles relating to good practice.

Anti-discriminatory/anti-bias practice means putting equal opportunities into action and this requires the examination of one's own values and expectations and readjusting these in order to ensure that, as a child care worker, one enables all children and their families to have equality of opportunity. Anti-discriminatory practice is not just related to race or colour but also refers to gender, lifestyles, class distinctions and ability/disability. There is good evidence that certain groups in society are discriminated against and therefore find it more difficult to get employment or decent housing; they find themselves living in areas that are poorly served by pre-school provision, health clinics or a good transport system.

Child care workers also need to be aware of the negative stereotypical images, which are depicted in the media, of ethnic minorities, women, people with disabilities and people who are poor. It is very damaging for children's self-esteem to grow up surrounded by negative images. Therefore it is important that resources used with children, such as videos, books, posters, toys and games, are carefully scrutinized to ensure that they do not contain negative stereotypes. There are organizations such as the Working Group Against Racism in Children's Resources, Letterbox Library and Early Years Trainers Anti-racist Network which are able to provide checklists, book lists and lists of suppliers to help child care workers select appropriate materials. (See also the list of organizations in the Appendix for addresses.)

Since the wars in Bosnia and Kosova and the alleged programmes of ethnic cleansing that have taken place in Eastern Europe there have been large numbers of refugees and asylum seekers coming to Britain. Although these people are seeking refuge in Britain there has been a very strong prejudicial movement against these groups, often from the people in the locality where they have been housed. Child care workers need to be aware that children in these families have probably had very traumatic experiences before they reached the UK and need careful, sensitive handling to help them rebuild their lives in a secure environment. They are also likely to have very little or no English language and this can be very frightening for small children, although given the right experiences and understanding they will very quickly learn the language from staff and other children.

The Hidden Curriculum

This is the name given to the social roles, gender roles, attitudes and values that are communicated to the child in ways other than through the curriculum: the unspoken lessons that children learn from other children and adults.

From a very early age, children are absorbing information from what they see and hear around them; stereotyping and labelling can

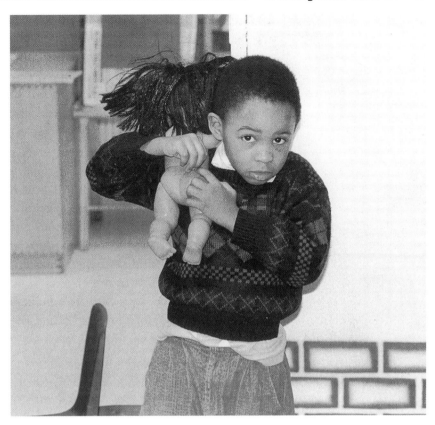

have a very damaging effect upon children. Making assumptions about children on the strength of how a previous member of the family behaved or how the child's parents behave, e.g. 'Well what can you expect of a child from that family, have you met the mother?' is very damaging to children and goes against good child care practice. Children who grow up feeling that they are inferior because of their colour, race, disability, or family background will not be able to reach their full potential.

Scapegoating and labelling

We live in a society that has a tendency to discriminate against certain groups: women, ethnic groups, people with disabilities, to name but a few. Blaming a particular group of people for our own misfortunes or things that are wrong in society is a form of scape-goating and is a very dangerous thing to do. Unfortunately, it is much easier to blame somebody else than to examine the situation and blame those who are really responsible, or undergo self-criticism in order to see where we have gone wrong. Most societies hold stereotypical views of one sort or another; for example, in Western society there is a stereotypical view that all scientists wear glasses and have white coats. How true is this? Researchers into this area have found that very few stereotypes are actually true represent-ations. The media are responsible for creating and perpetuating many stereotypes within our society. Stereotypes often come to the fore when dealing with parents: how influential upon a carer's atti-tude towards a parent is what the person may be wearing, the spoken accent, whether they arrive in a car or walk?

Labelling is a form of stereotyping but usually refers to giving certain attributes to a child or person, the attributes being based upon stereotypes. A lot of labelling can take place in staff rooms where it may not be uncommon to hear remarks such as, 'We have Sally Y starting at playgroup today. I should watch out for her, I had her sister last year and she was a real problem.' Poor Sally has no opportunity to show that she is different from her sister; she has been labelled before she even enters the building.

Rosenthal and Jacobson (1968) carried out a very famous experi-ment called 'Pygmalion in the Classroom', where they told teachers the names of the children who would be high fliers and those who would not be so able. At the end of the experimental period all the children had lived up to their label as either high fliers or less able, in spite of the fact that Rosenthal and Jacobson's choice had been arbitrary and was not based on any prior knowledge of the children. This experiment shows just how powerful the labelling system is and how it is able to influence the teacher's expectations of the chil-dren. These findings were upheld by the Swann Report (HMSO 1985) which found that teachers' low expectations were one of the main reasons for black children underachieving.

It is important that child care workers do not make assumptions about children or parents based upon dubious information. Many child care professionals have had the experience of thinking a child is the instigator of all the fights, only to find, when they have care-fully observed the situation, that in fact the other children were pro-voking the child. This is one of the very important uses of child observation techniques. It is very daunting for small children to have to prove that they are not as badly behaved as an older brother or sister, nor are they likely to behave in the same way as their out-spoken, aggressive parent. We all know that some children relate better to some members of staff and this can result in two staff members giving conflicting reports on how a child behaves. It is important that children are accepted on their face value and treated accordingly.

Gender issues

It is not unusual in our society to find females being treated differently from males. This happens in the wider society and may be reflected within the home or in the playgroup or other pre-school facility that the child attends. The Sex Discrimination Acts of 1975 and 1986 made it unlawful to discriminate against a person on the grounds of gender.

There is a large amount of research which shows that the early play experiences of girls are likely to result in them being less aware of space and less adept at large motor skills such as riding bicycles and using climbing frames. There is a tendency for child care workers to direct girls towards quiet activities, the home corner, the dressing up corner, the book corner etc. There is a tendency to direct boys towards the more boisterous activities such as bicycles, climbing frames, large building bricks, rough and tumble corners etc. If all children are to have equal access to all activities, with the staff giving all children equal encouragement to take part in these activities, then this must become a positive policy of the establishment rather than just left to the decision of each individual member of staff. The nursery or playgroup is the ideal place for children to experiment as it offers different experiences and opportunities which may not be available to them at home, for example boys being able to dress up or play with dolls.

Good practice in this area is reliant upon the attitudes of the staff and it is important that they do not discourage children from experimenting in this way. Staff need to be aware of the way in which they use language which can reinforce gender stereotypes. Expressions such as 'Boys do not cry', 'Girls should not climb trees', 'Boys do not dress up in girls' clothes', 'Girls do not play with trains' and 'What a tom-boy you are Sarah', only succeed in deterring children from experimenting. Sexist attitudes can be as damaging to boys as they are to girls. Not all boys want to climb trees, play boisterous games or ride bicycles. When children are playing in the hospital corner it is most common to find that the boys are the doctors and the girls are nurses, but it is the duty of the carers to ensure that each child is given a turn at being a doctor or a nurse.

It is also important for the nursery or playgroup to exhibit positive role models which are not gender specific, for example having books and stories about girls doing adventurous things and boys participating in caring activities, having pictures which show women driving buses, building houses, fighting fires etc. and men looking after children, preparing meals, nursing, caring for the elderly etc. Of course the ideal situation would be to have a mixed gender staff

SCENARIO 1.3

As a play group leader you have noticed that during outdoor play the boys take over all the bicycles and play aggressively, having mock shoot outs and mock fighting games. The girls and younger children are afraid of the boys. Describe how you would deal with this situation.

in the nursery and play group so that the male staff are able to offer positive role models to the children.

Race, colour and ethnicity

It has already been mentioned in this chapter that the UK is a pluralistic society. The population of the UK is made up of people from a wide variety of religious, racial and ethnic origins.

Immigration to the UK is not a new phenomenon; Peter Fryer (1984) records that the first black people arrived in Britain with the Roman army. In the 1800s there were large immigrations of Irish who were fleeing from the famine and Jews from Eastern Europe who were fleeing from the pogroms. The 1950s and 1960s saw immigrations of people from the West Indies, Asia and Africa. As the UK is a member of the European Union and there is now free movement between all 15 member states, it is likely that there will be more French, Germans, Dutch, Danes etc. living and working in the UK. The UK has a Race Relations Act (1976) which, among other things, makes it unlawful to discriminate against people on grounds of race. However, laws do not stop people from treating other people differently; such changes require individuals to alter their attitudes.

All child care establishments should reflect the diversity of the society in their equipment, reading materials, pictures, displays, stories, rhymes etc. The images around the nursery should be positive. If meals are served, menus should be varied in order to include foods such as pizzas, curries, tropical fruit, rice, stir-fry etc.

Staff need to be aware of the language they use and understand that the word 'black' is often used as a negative descriptor, e.g. blackleg, blackmail, black sheep.

Research by Milner (1983) and Maximé (1991) shows that children as young as 3 years of age understand differences in colour and are aware of the racial hierarchy. Children learn this by seeing and hearing the people around them treating black people differently. This results in black children having poor self-esteem and gravitating towards a peer group where there are other black children. Siraj-Blatchford (1994) says that the most common form of racism experienced by young children is name calling or negative references to their colour or language. Sadly, research carried out by Wright (1992) found that it was not only the children who behaved in a racist manner but also the staff in the nursery and primary schools in her study.

Disability

It is national policy wherever possible to include children with special needs within the mainstream facilities available for under-fives. The

Education Acts (1981, 1988 and 1993) and the Code of Practice (Department of Education 1994) have made it easier to include such children into mainstream schooling. Some children may have special needs which require adaptations in order for them to access the nursery or school, such as a child with spina bifida who uses a wheelchair; whereas another child may have special needs which require extra staff time and attention, such as a child with a language deficit or behavioural problems. It is possible for any child to be categorized as having special needs at some stage in their development, but with additional help they may be redesignated. For many children it is not always obvious to other children and adults that they may have a special need, such as those with sickle cell anaemia or cystic fibrosis, unlike those with conditions such as cerebral palsy or Down's syndrome.

Children with special needs are categorized as 'children in need' under the Children Act 1989. There has been controversy over this categorization as parents and experts argue that just because a child has a special need, it does not automatically mean that the child has needs that are not being met. However, the categorization does enable local authorities to give extra help and support to families that have pre-school children with special needs. This would enable the children to have a place in a nursery, nursery school or other pre-school provision, which is supplied and paid for by the local authority. It also enables the local authority to arrange any home adaptations which may be required or provide special equipment.

Children are always curious about each other and will ask questions about those children who appear to be different. Children's questions should be answered honestly and positive images of the child with disabilities must be promoted by the child care worker. Sadly, Micheline Mason (1993) says:

> We live in a system with a very rigid definition of who is valuable and who isn't ... The expectations [by society and individuals] of disabled people are lower than those of non-disabled people. Disabled children live in a system which has set up expectations of where the majority of young disabled people will eventually end up. Most people still expect disabled people to remain segregated for most of their lives.

If Mason is right then child care workers need to closely examine their expectations, values and attitudes in relation to children with disabilities. If children with disabilities are to be truly included into mainstream provision then this must take into account the importance of mainstream provision being able to offer an anti-biased equal opportunity environment. There must be positive role models and images of children and adults with disabilities; there must be stories that depict children with disabilities in 'heroic' positions. Children with disabilities must be encouraged to participate in all the activities in the nursery, playgroup or school. Staff must be careful not to be over-protective and should encourage children with disabilities to make decisions for themselves. It is also useful if adults with disabilities can participate in nursery activities to offer positive images to the staff and children. This may be achieved by the nursery or playgroup linking with local facilities for adults with disabilities and inviting them to become volunteers or visit the nursery to participate in activities.

THE ANTI-BIAS CURRICULUM AND GOOD PRACTICE

Providing an anti-bias curriculum will not in itself eliminate discrimination within a child care establishment. However, Siraj-Blatchford (1994) states that by removing the biases which are harmful or counter-productive, this aids the well being of the children and their families and is a positive start. Staff need to take a proactive approach, by listening to children, intervening when name calling or stereotyped ideas are being expressed and generally making it clear to children and parents that there are specific expressions and behaviours which are not acceptable within the nursery. All children need to feel equally valued and this can only be done by the worker considering the whole child, the whole curriculum and the whole environment. Staff need to look at themselves as individuals and as child care workers and examine the values and beliefs that they are transmitting to the children in their care.

Resources do not combat bias but they are tools to be used with the children and should therefore be carefully chosen to ensure that they reflect the anti-bias ethos of the establishment. Staff support and training may be necessary before an establishment can begin to look at its practice and devise a strategy for the future. Staff should work as a cohesive team, all working to the same anti-bias goals and able to share their experiences and use the expertise and advice of professionals. Equal opportunity policies are now common in most child care establishments but in themselves do not lead to good practice. Any policy needs to be discussed and written by the whole staff team so that there is ownership and commitment to its implementation. A policy is no good if it is not translated into the everyday practices of the workers. Along with policies there is a need to develop strategies: how will the staff deal with racist, sexist or other

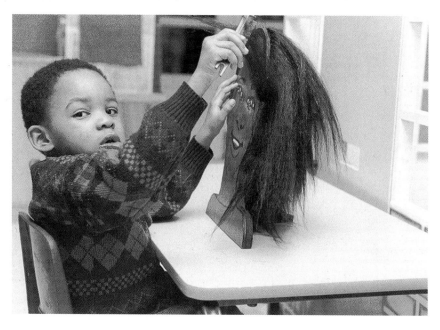

derogatory remarks that are made by the children? How will staff respond to children who refuse to sit next to a black child or a child who has disabilities or a child from a poor family who may not be wearing designer trainers? How will the staff ensure that all children are being valued as individuals? Derman-Sparks (1989) offers a checklist that staff can use to monitor their own good practice; the following is an adaptation of this:

- Do child care workers pick up on non-verbal and verbal expressions of interest as quickly with girls as they do with boys? With differently abled children? With black children?
- Do child care workers offer girls as much physical freedom and use of large motor equipment as they offer boys? Do they allow boys freedom to express feelings? Do they help more often or do more for girls than boys?
- Do child care workers provide adapted opportunities for children with certain limitations to interact actively and independently with materials and other children? Do they over-help or over-protect children who are different?
- Are similar behaviours interpreted and responded to differently with boys than with girls? White children than black children? Able bodied than differently abled children? For example do child care workers respond differently to an aggressive act of a boy or a black child or a child with special needs?

SCENARIO 1.4

The staff at your community nursery have decided to develop an anti-bias curriculum. As the senior worker it is your task to explain what this means to the Management Committee and to ask them to release the appropriate resources in order to put the idea into practice. Draw up a presentation for the Management Committee which clearly states the underlying principles of the anti-bias curriculum, the strategies for implementation and the resources that will be required.

Finally, Iram Siraj-Blatchford (1994) offer the following list that child care workers can use to ensure that they are offering an anti-racist curriculum:

The curriculum will:

- develop an understanding that people come from a range of backgrounds and cultures and offer children a secure environment in which to explore their own culture;
- offer opportunities for children to explore the idea that no culture, language or religion is more superior than others;
- depict a range of families;
- show people from a range of ethnic backgrounds doing everyday things;
- use the children's interests in planning, and to extend their learning;
- find appropriate resources and examples from a range of cultures for each topic over and above the everyday multicultural toys, poster etc;
- depict a range of child rearing practices from different cultures;
- help children talk about and challenge stereotyping;
- promote social and emotional development and teach about caring and sharing;
- involve parents and community groups in visiting and talking/working with children;
- illustrate through the curriculum that human achievements are universal and not just Western;
- expect high standards of achievement from all the children.

ASSIGNMENTS

1. Write an essay on the advantages and disadvantages of living in an extended family.

2. What effects does poverty have on the lives of family members?

3. What do you understand by bed-and-breakfast accommodation? What are the possible effects that bed-and-breakfast accommodation could have on a child's development?

4. 'Poverty is a phenomenon of the lower social classes'. Discuss this statement.

5. What do you understand by the term 'anti-bias practice'? What checks could you use to audit a setting in order to monitor the implementation of anti-bias practice?

6. You overhear Raymond (aged 5 years) calling Peter (aged 4 years) a 'spastic'. What action, if any, do you take?

7. You overhear a member of staff telling Sally (aged 4 years) that girls do not climb trees. What action, if any, do you take?

8. What do you understand by the term 'hidden curriculum'?

PRACTICAL ACTIVITIES

1. Carry out an audit of the setting where you work or are on placement and answer the following questions:
   a) What alterations, if any, would need to be made to enable a wheelchair user to gain access to your setting?
   b) What, if any, mobility problems may the setting present to a child who is partially sighted?

2. Observe a small group of children aged 3–5 years in the outdoor play area. Choose one boy and one girl. Note the length of time the girl spends on the climbing frame and the bicycle. Note the length of time the girl spends with the doll's pram. Note the length of time the boy spends on the climbing frame and the bicycle. Note the length of time the boy spends with the doll's pram. Write up conclusions to your findings and discuss the outcomes with your placement supervisor or tutor.

3. Observe a small group of 4–5 year olds playing in the home corner and record their conversations. Does anything in their conversation or actions offer insights into gender stereotyping?

4. Draw up a list of books suitable for 3–5 year olds which are relevant to the following:
   a) Show positive images of child/children with disabilities
   b) Depict children in a non-nuclear family situation
   c) Depict children in a pluralistic society
   d) Offer a traditional story from a particular culture.

References

Bradshaw J 1990 Child poverty and deprivation in the UK. National Children's Bureau, London

Burgoyne J, Clark D 1982 Reconstituted families. In: Rapoport RN, Fogarty MP, Rapoport R (eds) Families in Britain. Routledge & Kegan Paul, London

Calouste Gulbenkian Foundation 1995 Children and violence: report of the commission on children and violence. Calouste Gulbenkian Foundation, London

Department of Education 1994 Code of practice on the identification and assessment of special educational need. HMSO, London

Derman-Sparks L 1989 Anti-bias curriculum: tools for empowering young children. National Association for the Education of Young Children, Washington DC, p8

Fryer P 1984 Staying power: the history of black people in Britain. Pluto Press, London

HMSO 1985 Education for all. The Swann report. HMSO, London

HMSO 1999 Opportunity for all: tackling poverty and social exclusion. HMSO Cm 4445, London

Kumar V 1993 Poverty and inequality in the UK: the effect on children. National Children's Bureau, London

Mason M 1993 Disability bias. Co-ordinate 33:13–14

Maximé JE 1991 Towards a transcultural approach to working with under sevens. In: Report of two conferences combating racism among students, staff and children. NCB/EYARN, London

Milner D 1983 Children and race: 10 years on. Ward Lock Educational, London

Moss P 1988 Childcare and equality of opportunity. European Commission, Brussels

Newsom J, Newsom E 1976 Seven years old in the home environment. Allen & Unwin, London

Oppenheim C 1993 Poverty: the facts. Child Poverty Action Group, London

Rosenthal R, Jacobson L 1968 Pygmalion in the classroom. Rosehart & Winston, New York

Siraj-Blatchford I 1994 The early years: laying the foundations for racial equality. Trentham Books, London

Tizard B, Blatchford P, Burke J, Farquhor C, Plewis I 1988 Young children at school in the inner city. Lawrence Erlbaum Associates, London

Wright C 1992 Early education: multicultural primary school classrooms. In: Gill D (ed) Racism and education. Sage, London

Young M, Wilmott P 1962 Family and kinship in East London. Penguin Books, Harmondsworth

Further reading

■ Andreski R, Nicholls S 1995 Setting standards: a guide for the nursery professional. Nursery World, London

■ Aspinwall K 1984 What are little girls made of? What are little boys made of? NNEB, St Albans

■ Braun D 1992 Working with parents. In: Pugh G (ed) Contemporary issues in the early years. Paul Chapman/NCB, London

■ Browne N 1993 Girls and boys go out to play. Childcare Now 13(1):20

■ Browne N, France P 1986 Untying the apron strings: anti-sexist provision for the under fives. Open University Press, Milton Keynes

■ Cameron C, Moss P, Owen C 1999 Men in the nursery: gender and caring work. Paul Chapman, London

■ Candappa M 1995 Equal opportunities and ethnicity in early childhood services. Childcare Now 15(3):10

■ Cochran M, Larner M, Riley D, Gunnarsson L, Henderson C 1993 Extending families: the social networks of parents and their children. Cambridge University Press, Cambridge

■ Commission for Racial Equality 1996 From cradle to school. A practical guide to racial equality in early childhood education and care, revised edn. Commission for Racial Equality, London

■ Derman-Sparks L 1993 How to challenge bias in childcare. Co-ordinate 33 (January):8

■ Dixon B 1990 Playing them false: a study of children's toys, games and puzzles. Trentham Books, Staffordshire

- Drummond MJ 1993 Learning about gender bias. Co-ordinate 33(January):17

- Elfer P 1995 With equal concern? National Children's Bureau, London

- Equal Opportunities Commission 1995 An equal start. Guidelines on equal treatment for the under eights. Equal Opportunities Commission, Cardiff

- Grabrucker M 1988 There's a good girl: gender stereotyping in the first three years of life: a diary. The Women's Press, London

- Kenway P, Hyder T 1995 Offering children an equal start. Co-ordinate 45(January):4

- Lane J 1995 No equality no quality. Childcare Now 15(3):8

- Lane J 1999 Action for racial equality in the early years. The National Early Years Network, London

- Leach P 1994 Children first. Michael Joseph, London

- Millam R 1996 Anti-discriminatory practice: a guide for workers in childcare and education. Cassells, London

- Phillips A 1993 The trouble with boys: parenting the men of the future. Pandora, London

- Potts P 1993 Learning for all. Childcare Now 13(1):9

- Pre-school Playgroup Association 1991 Equal chances: eliminating discrimination and ensuring equality of opportunity in playgroups. PPA, London

- Reiser R, Mason M 1990 Disability equality in the classroom: a human rights issue. Inner London Education Authority, London (Available from: Disability Equality in Education, 78 Mildmay Grove, London N1 4PJ)

- Robson B 1989 Pre-school provision for children with special needs. Cassells, London

- Siencyn SW 1993 Bilingual start for young Welsh. Childcare Now 13(1):9

- Slaby R, Roedell W, Arezzo D, Hendrix K 1995 Early violence prevention: tools for teachers of young children. National Association for the Education of Young Children, Washington DC (Available in UK from Early Years Training Network, (formerly VOLCUF))

- Sudbury J 1993 Challenging racism in the early years. Childcare Now 13(1):15

- Troyna B, Hatcher R 1992 Racism in children's lives. Routledge/NCB, London

- Twitchin J 1988 The black and white media show book. Handbook for the study of racism and television. Trentham Books, Staffordshire

- Wolfendale S (ed) 2000 Special needs in the early years: snapshots of practice. Routledge, London

- Wolfendale S, Wooster J 1992 Meeting special needs in the early years. In: Pugh G (ed) Contemporary issues in the early years. Paul Chapman/NCB, London

Chapter 2

Child Health

This chapter covers underpinning knowledge for all or parts of the following units for the National Vocational Qualifications (NVQs) in Early Years Care and Education: C1, C2. It is also linked to the following CACHE Awards Units: Diploma Units 3, 5; Certificate Unit 1.

INTRODUCTION

If children are to be kept safe from disease and illness it is important that the child care worker has a good grasp of the underlying principles of health. Child care workers have a responsibility to ensure that the children in their care are able to enjoy their developmental experiences and activities without being exposed to undue risks in the environment. Part of this responsibility involves child care workers carrying out measures in their daily activities in order to prevent primary infection or the spread of disease to the children in their care. Child care workers must have a high standard of personal hygiene.

In the Victorian era, diseases such as tuberculosis were common and quickly spread through a population which had poor diet, poor washing facilities, poorly heated accommodation and dubious personal hygiene. Present day living conditions and our greater knowledge of how diseases are spread go a long way to preventing the outbreak of epidemics within society.

The World Health Organization (WHO) defines the following factors as essential to the health and development of children:

- Food and drink in sufficient quantity and nutritionally adequate
- Warmth
- Fresh air
- Exercise
- Rest and sleep
- Good posture
- Personal and communal health
- Dental care
- Sensible clothing
- Prevention of illness and injury
- Medical supervision.

The responsibility for ensuring that children receive the above basic needs rests with the government, individual families and carers.

MULTI-CULTURAL ASPECTS OF CHILDREN'S ILLNESSES

Throughout this chapter there will be descriptions of signs and symptoms of common childhood ailments. It must be noted that these descriptions only apply to white skin. In children who have brown or black skin tones, rashes will look different from the descriptions given here; for example, on a black skin a rash will not look red, although it will still be raised or have vesicles. It should also be noted that where reference is made to skin pallor again this refers to white skin. Children with black or brown skin do go pale when they are sick, however, this is not always as obvious as it is in white skin; in fact the child may look greyish. Parents and carers who are familiar with the child will be able to recognize skin pallor in a black child but it may not be so obvious to others. If a black child is having difficulty in breathing any blueness of the skin may be difficult to detect, therefore there is a need to check the child's lips and fingernails. If these are showing signs of blueness then this will denote cyanosis which indicates a serious breathing problem requiring immediate emergency treatment.

INFECTIONS

All disease is caused by germs, a generic term to describe three types of infection: bacterial, fungal and viral (Box 2.1). Once germs have established themselves in a favourable situation they have a very fast breeding rate, some doubling their numbers every half hour. The period when the organisms are multiplying but the body is not showing any symptoms of the disease is called the incubation period.

Box 2.1 *Common infectious diseases of childhood*

Disease: Common cold (Coryza)
Incubation period: 1–3 days
Cause: Virus
Method of spread: Airborne, but can also be spread by hands through infected person touching eyes, mouth and nose, and hence carrying pathogens in secretions
Signs and symptoms: Sneezing, sore throat, stuffy nose, running nose; headache, partial deafness; slight rise in temperature (pyrexia), child irritable, not interested in play
Complications: Sinusitis, laryngitis, tracheitis, bronchitis
Treatment: No specific cure; symptoms treated; comfort and hot drinks; junior paracetamol if prescribed by doctor; vaseline or other oil based cream applied to nostrils to prevent soreness due to discharge

Box 2.1 *continued*

First day   Third day
of rash   of rash

Disease: Chickenpox (*Varicella*)
Incubation period: 2 weeks
Cause: Virus
Method of spread: Airborne (and by discharge from skin lesions)
Signs and symptoms: Mild onset – off colour, slight pyrexia; rash appears first on trunk, then face, then limbs; lesions are little vesicles (blisters) surrounded by a ring of inflammation; blisters can erupt easily; vesicles become filled with pus (pustules) then dry up to form scabs; rash appears in crops so three stages (vesicles, pustules and scabs) may all be seen at one time; child will feel ill, with severe headache, and find spots irritating
Complications: Scarring and secondary infection only if there is scratching of spots
Treatment: Calamine lotion is soothing for irritation; relief of other symptoms; particular care of skin to prevent chafing and complications; child's nails should be cut short to prevent secondary infection through scratching, gloves applied if itching is severe; if lesions are profuse penicillin may be prescribed to prevent secondary infection

Disease: Measles (less common since vaccinations became available)
Incubation period: 1–2 weeks
Cause: Virus
Method of spread: Airborne
Signs and symptoms: Running nose, watery eyes, fever, cough; Koplik's spots – red with white centres – may be seen inside the mouth in 1 or 2 days then disappear; 3rd day fever subsides; 4th day temperature rises again maybe as high as 104°F as rash appears; blotchy red rash spreads down over the body from the face; child fretful, irritable, hot, with cough and painful eyes
Complications: Otitis media (middle ear infection), pneumonia, corneal ulceration (rare), encephalitis (rare)
Treatment: Requires special attention. Drugs may be prescribed to prevent complications; relief of symptoms; bedroom/sickroom shaded if photophobia (sensitive to light) present; attention to diet as vomiting may occur; plenty of fluids; convalescence in fresh air and sunshine

Disease: Mumps (epidemic parotitis) (less common since vaccinations became available)
Incubation period: 2–3 weeks
Cause: Virus
Method of spread: Airborne
Signs and symptoms: General malaise, pain and swelling of parotid glands (in front of and under the ear) on one or both sides of the face; rise in temperature, sore throat, headache may develop before glands swell; flow of saliva may increase or

Box 2.1 *continued*

diminish – affects feeding; jaws painful – patient may refuse feed or find difficulty in chewing
Complications: Meningitis (rare), orchitis (inflammation of testes, usually only in adolescent boys, rarely causes sterility)
Treatment: No specific cure; care of mouth – cleanliness and moistness; plenty of fluids, through a straw (which has a good effect on the child who may be feeling miserable and will enjoy departure from normal methods of drinking)

Disease: Whooping cough (pertussis) (less common since vaccinations became available)
Incubation period: 1–2 weeks
Cause: Bacillus
Method of spread: Airborne
Signs and symptoms: Affects mainly children under five; cough usually first symptom often accompanied by clear, watery, nasal discharge. Coughing becomes more frequent then paroxysmal and temperature rises; whoop follows a number of short, sharp, expiratory coughs; the cough reflex closes the glottis and the child cannot take a breath until the outburst is over: thus he appears to be suffocating – may turn blue, red or purple, eyes seem enlarged and protruding; drawing in air against the resistance of the glottis causes whoop. Production of thick mucus and vomiting usually follows the cough; paroxysms of coughing may leave the child exhausted; babies do not usually acquire whooping cough
Complications: Otitis media, bronchopneumonia, convulsions in babies under 1 year old – may lead to brain damage
Treatment: Requires extra special attention. Coughing may continue for several weeks; the child may be reluctant to have feed because of vomiting; paroxysms are less frequent after 2–3 weeks and temperature is usually normal in about 2 months. Child must be kept warm, moist inhalations can be given and linctus may be prescribed for the cough; antibiotics may be prescribed to prevent complications in the chest. Support and comfort should be given during paroxysms which are frightening; a feed may be given after an attack to give time for absorption before the next coughing fit

First day of rash   Third day of rash

Disease: Rubella (German measles) (less common since vaccinations became available)
Incubation period: 2–3 weeks
Cause: Virus
Method of spread: Airborne
Signs and symptoms: Mild symptoms – headache, stiff neck, running nose, rash of pink spots behind the ears and forehead, may be swollen glands at back of neck; child may feel unwell

Box 2.1 *continued*

First day
of rash

Third day
of rash

Complications: Only if contracted by women in first 3 months of pregnancy – baby may be born with deafness, heart abnormalities and general malformations
Treatment: Treat symptoms

Disease: Scarlet fever (scarlatina) (rare now in Europe)
Incubation period: 2–7 days
Notifiable disease
Cause: Bacillus
Method of spread: Droplet infection
Signs and symptoms: Sore throat, swollen lymph glands in the neck, tonsils may be covered with purulent discharge, bright red rash appears on second day lasting 2–3 days, with flaking of skin over area of rash, especially on palms and soles of feet
Complications: Uncommon
Treatment: Isolation, antibiotics, treat symptoms

Disease: Dysentery (means inflammation of colon and rectum; can be caused by amoebae or bacilli, but bacillary type most common in UK)
Incubation period: 1–7 days (usually 3–4 days)
Cause: Bacillus
Method of spread: Excreted in stools so spread through poor sanitation, poor sewage disposal and by lack of hand-washing. Spread in food
Signs and symptoms: Diarrhoea often with blood and mucus; fever, headache, muscular pain; diagnosis made by taking specimen of stools, or from a rectal swab
Complications: Shock and prostration, dehydration through loss of fluid and salts; can be fatal, particularly in young children and babies
Treatment: Isolation; excreta disposed of only after disinfecting; fluid or low-residue diet, i.e. foods which are easily digested such as fruit purees, jellies, thickened soups, eggs, minced meat and fish, ice-cream. Drugs as prescribed by the doctor. Three negative swabs required before patient is pronounced cured. Strict hygiene in food handling. Important that child is given plenty of fluids

Disease: Gastroenteritis (infantile)
Cause: *Escherichia coli*, *Salmonella* or dysentery bacillus, viral infection or secondary to other infection, e.g. otitis media
Method of spread: Rare in breast fed babies
Signs and symptoms: Looser bowel action sometimes with blood or mucus or coloured green or bright orange; occasional vomiting and rejection of feeds despite obvious thirst and hunger. Reduced urinary output, weight loss, dehydration; restlessness and general malaise

Box 2.1 *continued*

Complications: Dehydration often rapid and severe with metabolic and electrolyte disturbances; these, if uncorrected, can lead to convulsions, renal failure and death

Treatment: Requires special attention. Give child plenty of fluids such as plain cooled boiled water

Disease: Meningitis

Incubation period: 2–10 days but can be variable

Cause: Bacterial meningitis, of which there are two main types: meningococcal and pneumococcal. Haemophilus influenza type b (Hib) which was a major cause of bacterial meningitis has now been almost eliminated by vaccination of infants. Viral meningitis is caused most commonly by the coxsackie virus and the echovirus (also known as enterovirus). Meningitis can also develop as a result of infection with herpes simplex, measles, polio or chickenpox

Method of spread: Airborne or droplet

Signs and symptoms: In babies: high temperature, fever with cold hands and feet; vomiting or refusal to eat; high pitched moaning, whimpering cry, blank staring expression, pale blotchy complexion; baby may be floppy, may dislike being handled and may be fretful, difficult to wake up or lethargic; the fontanelle (soft spot on babies' heads) may be tense or bulging. In children and adults: high temperature, fever, possibly cold hands and feet, vomiting, sometimes diarrhoea; severe headache, neck stiffness (unable to touch the chin to the chest), joint or muscle pains; sometimes stomach cramps with septicaemia; dislike of bright lights, drowsiness, having fits, confusion or disorientation

Both adults and children may have a rash (septicaemic rash) which may start anywhere on the body as a cluster of tiny blood spots, which look like pin-pricks in the skin. If untreated these blood spots will join to give the appearance of fresh bruises. The 'glass test' can be used to see if a rash might be septicaemia. If you press the side of a clear drinking glass firmly onto the spots or bruises they will not fade. Do not wait for the rash before seeking medical advice as it may be the last symptom to appear and in cases of meningitis without septicaemia it may never appear

Complications: Brain damage (1:7 survivors are left with serious disability), death (fatal in 1:10 cases)

Treatment: Viral meningitis cannot be helped by antibiotics and treatment is by good nursing care. Bacterial meningitis requires immediate medical treatment with antibiotics; the sooner the disease is diagnosed and treated the greater the chance of the child making a full recovery

Bacteria

These are microorganisms which are made up of a single cell. They are not all harmful to the body, in fact a number of bacteria live in the gut and aid the digestive processes. Harmful bacteria produce toxins which are not able to be neutralized by the body's natural defence mechanisms (called antibodies) and this results in illness. Bacterial infections can be treated with antibiotics, although overuse of antibiotics has led to some bacteria becoming resistant to them. Examples of harmful bacteria are *Streptococcus*, which causes sore throats, scarlet fever; *Staphylococcus*, which causes boils, styes etc; *Diplococcus*, which causes pneumonia, meningitis (bacterial type) etc.; bacilli, which cause tuberculosis, typhoid etc.

Fungi

These are plants which do not have chlorophyll and feed on dead or living organic matter. They are the same family as mushrooms, toadstools, moulds and lichens. Those that live on or in the human body are much smaller and often cannot be seen without a microscope. The most common illnesses caused by fungal infections are thrush and athlete's foot. Fungal infections are easily treated with anti-fungal medications. They do not require treatment with antibiotics.

Viruses

These are very small microorganisms which operate in a complex way by invading the cells of the body and altering the way that the cell behaves. They cause illnesses such as mumps, measles, influenza, polio etc. In general they are not treatable with antibiotics, but the body is able to build its resistance to common viral infections by immunization.

INFESTATIONS

This is the term used to describe the situation where parasites live on or inside the body. Parasites may be head lice, body lice, thread worms, tape worm etc.

SCENARIO 2.1

Jasmine is a childminder and one of the children that she cares for is Sian aged 2 years. Today Sian seems unwell: she has a rise in her temperature, a runny nose, watery eyes and looks generally unwell. When Jasmine examines her she looks in her mouth and finds that Sian has small white spots like breadcrumbs inside her mouth. What do you think is wrong with Sian? What action will Jasmine need to take?

SPREAD OF INFECTION

There are four main routes by which infection is able to enter the body:

1. *Inhalation* – the organism is breathed out by an infectious person and then inhaled by the next person who will then become infected. Examples of illnesses passed on in this way are the viral diseases influenza and measles.

2. *Ingestion* – the person becomes infected by eating contaminated food or drinking contaminated water. Illnesses spread in this way are, e.g. salmonella poisoning, typhoid.

3. *Inoculation* – the organism gains access to the body through a wound in the skin, or the bite of an insect. Illnesses spread in this way are, e.g. malaria and post-operative wound infections.

4. Very rarely, infection can be transmitted before a child is born, via the placenta or the mother's blood supply. Examples of such illnesses are syphilis, AIDS/HIV.

People come into contact with infection through a number of ways:

1. *Carriers* – people who have no symptoms of the disease but who are still able to pass the disease on to other people. They may be people who have had the disease and are now in the convalescent stage. A person is unaware that they are the 'carrier' of a disease. The most famous 'carrier' was a woman known as 'Typhoid Annie' who was thought to have been responsible for a widespread typhoid epidemic which took place in the United States during the nineteenth century.

Another type of carrier is called a vector. This is when an organism passes on a parasite, for example the mosquito transmits the malaria parasite. Household pets such as cats, dogs and birds act as vectors and can pass worms and fleas on to children.

2. *Direct spread* – through bodily contact with the infected person. Illnesses which are passed on by direct contact are referred to as being contagious. Examples of these are impetigo and some forms of conjunctivitis.

3. *Indirect spread* – through the handling of infected objects such as dressings or contaminated faeces. In other cases contaminated food or water may lead to the indirect spread of diseases such as salmonella poisoning, typhoid and cholera. The contamination may have reached the food via flies, which are known to be responsible for the spread of dysentery, gastroenteritis, influenza and poliomyelitis.

4. *Airborne or droplet spread* – minute droplets from the nose and mouth of an infected person are spread by sneezing, or dry out and

are then spread by the air. Illnesses spread in this way are the common cold, respiratory tract infections, measles, mumps, chicken-pox and other common childhood illnesses.

THE BODY'S DEFENCES AGAINST INFECTION

The body has a number of ways of defending itself against infection. Externally, the skin has a protective function, as do the tear ducts in eyes and the mucous membrane in the nose. The nasal passages also have tiny hairs (cilia) which line the nose and act as filter mechanisms for germs.

Internally, the body has a lymphatic system which consists of a series of lymph glands connected by lymphatic vessels (tubes). The lymph nodes (glands) produce lymphocytes which are capable of destroying foreign antigens and of producing antibodies. These are part of the body's immune response to infection. Lymph nodes also act as filters for infection; the tonsils are lymph nodes.

The white blood cells (leucocytes and phagocytes) fight infection by producing an immune response in the body. When infection is present the number of leucocytes present in the blood is increased.

Antibodies are proteins formed in the spleen or lymph nodes which are produced as a response to the antigens of invading bacteria. Antibodies can be produced by a person actually having the illness and therefore becoming immune to contracting the same disease again, for example in measles. They can also be triggered off by the introduction into the body of antigens; this is how a number of immunization vaccines work. Thus the measles vaccine will introduce a mild form of measles antigen into the body which will then produce antibodies to offer the person immunity against measles; this is called acquired immunity.

Antitoxins are a type of antibody which neutralize toxins that are formed in the blood by certain types of bacteria. As with antibodies, they can be produced by a person having the illness or they can be artificially introduced by the injection of a weak strain of the toxin, as in the case of tetanus.

TYPES OF IMMUNITY

Immunity is the power of resisting infection due to the effects of antibodies and antitoxins. There are two types of immunity, active and passive.

Active Immunity

This is the way the body responds to the antigens and toxins produced by bacteria or other types of infection. There are two types of active immunity, natural and artificial.

Natural active immunity	This is when immunity has been acquired through: 1. Actually having an attack of the disease and producing antibodies which give lifelong immunity, e.g. measles, rubella 2. Having a mild attack of the illness which may show very few symptoms but which does invade the body's defences enough to produce antibodies. Repeated mild attacks of an illness will produce the same effects.
Artificial active immunity	This is when immunity is acquired through inoculation with: 1. Living organisms, e.g. smallpox vaccine 2. Living weakened organisms, e.g. BCG (Bacillus Calmette-Guerin), tuberculosis vaccine 3. Dead organisms, e.g. whooping cough (pertussis) vaccine 4. Modified toxins (toxoid), e.g. diphtheria vaccine.
Passive Immunity	This may be acquired naturally or artificially.
Natural passive immunity	This is the immunity which a baby obtains from its mother. Part of this immunity would have been passed to the child whilst it was still in the womb, via the placenta. Additional immunity is passed to the child via the mother's milk; this is why breast feeding is so important, particularly in those early days following the birth.
Artificial passive immunity	This offers temporary protection from a disease by injecting serum from a person or animal. The effects will only last 3–4 weeks, as once the antibodies die out, so will the immunity. It is not used very often as it only has a short term effect.
IMMUNIZATION	Before the discovery of vaccines, many children died from the common childhood illnesses such as diphtheria, whooping cough (pertussis) and smallpox. Even today, in countries where there is no comprehensive child immunization programme, children still die or are left permanently damaged due to contracting common childhood illnesses. Although there has been negative publicity given on the side effects of some types of immunization, particularly the link between whooping cough (pertussis) vaccine and brain damage, the dangers of the diseases are much greater than the small risks associated with children being immunized.

The reasons for immunizing children are:

- Some infectious diseases are extremely dangerous and can be fatal in children under 1 year, e.g. whooping cough (pertussis)
- Complications of infectious diseases may cause handicaps or disability, e.g. poliomyelitis can cause permanent paralysis, measles can affect eyesight and hearing
- Complications from infectious diseases can also affect the child's intellectual development, e.g. convulsions leading to brain damage (a complication of whooping cough (pertussis))
- Immunization reduces the number of people who will contract the disease and eventually this can eliminate the disease within society, e.g. the World Health Organization (WHO) now classes smallpox as having been eradicated.

Table 2.1
Immunization schedule[a]

Immunization	Age
BCG	Birth (for those at risk)
Triple vaccine (DTP)[b], polio and Hib[c]	8 weeks (1st) 12 weeks (2nd) 16 weeks (3rd)
Measles, mumps, rubella (MMR)	12–18 months[d]
Booster (diphtheria, tetanus and polio)	4–5 years
Rubella (girls only)	10–14 years
BCG (tuberculosis–tuberculin-negative children)	10–14 years[e] or infancy
Booster (tetanus and polio)	15–18 years

From the year 2000 there has been a new vaccine for children which offers protection from Meningitis type C. Children aged 1–5 years are able to be vaccinated via their general practitioner service whilst the 5–14 years age group are able to be vaccinated via the school health service. Babies are able to get this vaccine at the same time that they are getting the other immunizations i.e. at 2, 3 and 4 months and older infants are able to get it with the MMR. However, experts are pointing out that the vaccine will only protect children from one type of meningitis so that parents and carers still need to be alert for symptoms of other types of meningitis.
[a] Based on recommendations from a pamphlet issued by the Department of Health (1990) but with recent amendments added
[b] Diphtheria, tetanus and pertussis (whooping cough)
[c] From October 1992 Hib has been offered to all children under 4 years of age
[d] May be given at any age over 12 months
[e] Interval of 3 weeks between BCG and rubella

Child care workers should ensure that their own vaccinations are up-to-date as part of their duty of care to those children with whom they are working. There are some religious groups who object to immunization and will not allow their children to be vaccinated. As in all other decisions, the parents' or primary carers' wishes in these matters are to be respected. In the event of such a decision placing the child at risk then social services are able to apply to the courts for a ruling on what action can be taken.

Table 2.1 shows the immunization schedule for babies and children.

PREVENTION OF THE SPREAD OF INFECTION

Diet, fresh air and exercise all go towards preventing the spread of infection. In addition to these there are a number of practices which the child care worker needs to carry out as a matter of routine when dealing with children and these can be found in the following hygiene procedures put forward by the Department of Health (1992), which, although written for those who deal with HIV positive children, are good practice for all situations.

Hygiene Procedures

1. The following hygiene procedures are recommended as safe practice for all staff and all those who care for children whether in private homes or group settings. The procedures should not be limited to those knowingly involved in the care of children with HIV. These are common sense precautions which will protect against a range of minor and major infection which may be transmitted via blood and body fluids...

General measures

2. Cuts or sores which break the skin on the hands should be kept covered with waterproof adhesive or other suitable dressing.

3. Hands should be washed thoroughly:

   - before and after carrying out First Aid procedures involving external bleeding and/or broken skin
   - after contact with blood or body fluids (semen, faeces, urine or vomit).

4. Where possible, disposable gloves should be used when carrying out First Aid. Household rubber gloves should always be used if heavily soiled material, or bleach, is being handled. It is important to ensure the safe storage of bleach in areas which involve children and to which children have access.

5. Razor blades, toothbrushes etc. which may be contaminated with blood should not be shared. (Needles etc. used for intravenous therapy at home should be stored/disposed of in appropriate containers supplied by the Health Service. The

same safety precautions will apply to injecting equipment used for any other purposes, e.g. where someone has an injecting drug habit. They should be encouraged to take all the necessary safety precautions to prevent 'sharp' injuries to others including children.)

Accidents involving blood

6. Normal First Aid procedures should be followed, and should include the use of disposable gloves where possible. The wound should be washed immediately, squeezing to expel blood and using plenty of soap and water, and a suitable dressing applied or pressure pad if needed. Medical advice should be sought as soon as possible.

7. If blood is splashed onto the skin it should be washed off immediately with soap and water. Splashes of blood into the eyes or mouth should be washed out immediately with plenty of water.

8. After accidents resulting in bleeding, surfaces with blood on them, e.g. tables or furniture, should be cleaned liberally with household bleach, freshly diluted 1 in 10, that is 1 volume (e.g. cupful) of bleach should be added to 9 volumes (cupfuls) of water to make the required (effective) 1 in 10 solution. Alternatively, hot soapy water may be used. Bleach can corrode metal and burn holes in fabrics if used for too long or in the wrong concentration, and must never be used on the skin.

Cleaning

9. Normal cleaning methods should be used. No special disinfectants are necessary for either bath or toilet. Disposable cloths should be used, with a separate one for the kitchen, for the bathroom and for the toilet.

10. Spillage of blood, vomit and body fluids should be cleaned up as soon as possible. Ordinary domestic bleach, diluted 1 part in 10 parts with water, or hot soapy water, should be poured gently over the spill which has been covered with paper towels. If possible and convenient the diluted bleach should be left for 30 minutes. It should then be wiped up with disposable paper towels. More solid spillages, such as vomit or faeces, can be scooped up in a bucket of hot soapy water and the scoop cleaned or disposed of as contaminated waste.

11. Paper towels should be treated as infected waste. Disposable gloves and aprons should be thrown away as infected waste.

12. Clothing and linen (e.g. terry nappies, sheets, towels) which have been soiled with blood or body fluids should be washed in a well maintained washing machine, rinsing initially in the cold rinse cycle and then washing in the hot wash cycle (approximately 80 degrees centigrade). Overloading should be avoided. If handwashing is unavoidable, household rubber gloves must be worn and the water and detergent must be as hot as can be tolerated and the articles rinsed in hot water.

13. Crockery and cutlery can be cleaned by handwashing with hot soapy water or in a dishwasher or dish sterilizer.

Disposal of waste

14. Items which have been soiled with blood or body fluids may be flushed down the toilet if disposable (e.g. tampons) or burnt (e.g. paper towels, disposable nappies, sanitary towels). If this cannot be done on site, the rubbish, including protective disposable gloves or aprons, should be 'double bagged' in plastic bags and effectively secured. Arrangements should be made with the local authority for collection of this infected waste for incineration. Vomit, urine and faeces should be flushed down the toilet and potties should be washed with detergent or anti-septic and hot water and dried with paper towels.

(Department of Health 1992, with permission)

In addition to the Department of Health recommendations the following practices should also be carried out as part of the basic routine:

- Always wash your hands before handling food.
- Always wash your hands after using the toilet or helping a child to use the toilet.
- Always wash your hands before touching a baby or making up a baby's feed.
- Ensure that bathrooms, toilets and baby changing areas are cleaned/disinfected frequently and at least daily.
- Report to the parent or officer in charge any child with abnormal stools, high temperature or other sign of infection.
- Only use disposable handkerchiefs and ensure that, once used, they are kept away from the reach of children.
- Encourage and teach children to wash their hands after using the toilet and before meals.
- Be familiar with the establishment's policy for dealing with diarrhoea and other gastrointestinal infections.

- Ensure that each child has their own flannel, towel, toothbrush and hair brush, and that these are washed/disinfected frequently.
- Any cuts or open wounds on the hands should always be covered when dealing with children or food, or rubber gloves should be worn.
- Toys and other playthings should be washed/disinfected regularly, particularly soft toys.
- Ensure that children always wash their hands after playing with pets and do not let animals lick children's faces or hands.
- Ensure that all pets are free from worms or fleas and that hutches and tanks etc. are cleaned regularly.

SIGNS OF ILLNESS IN CHILDREN

How do you know when a child is feeling ill? There are a number of physical and behavioural signs that will alert the adult to sickness in a child. The child may feel hot, look flushed and have a raised temperature. There may be vomiting, diarrhoea or both. Children may complain of pain or that a part of them is hurting. They may become breathless or have difficulty in breathing. They may lose their appetite and refuse to eat or drink. They may look pale, with dark rings around their eyes. They may have constipation or difficulty in passing urine. They may have a rash or some other type of skin irritation. In addition to the physical signs there may also be changes in their behaviour. They may be fretful and crying or may become listless and withdrawn. They may cling to their parent or carer, not wanting to leave them or join in activities with the other children. They may be sleepy and not want to wake up after their afternoon nap. They may regress and forget their toilet training or only want to play with toys suitable for a younger age group. They may just generally not seem to be their normal selves.

DEALING WITH A SICK CHILD

If you are responsible for a child that becomes sick there are a number of important steps to take. First you need to ascertain whether the situation is an immediate emergency; for example, any difficulty in breathing, loss of consciousness or a convulsion (fit) would require immediate medical treatment. It is important to inform your superiors and/or the child's parents about the situation. The child should be made comfortable, resting in a quiet place with his favourite toy. The child will need to be reassured as he may be very frightened. You should make a note of any symptoms to give to the parents/doctor. If the child is vomiting or has diarrhoea, try to give him sips of water. Do not give any medicines unless they have been prescribed by a doctor. If the child has a very high temperature you should try to bring this down by tepid sponging and putting an electric fan in the room. A sick child should not be left alone.

COMMON CHILDHOOD ILLNESSES

This section looks at illnesses that are likely to be encountered by the child care worker. There is not room in this book to cite every likely illness that affects children; however, what is given is a selection of the most common. Some of the illnesses cited are minor and others are more serious and have long lasting effects on the child's lifestyle. The illnesses are in alphabetical order to make it simpler for the reader to find a reference quickly.

Asthma

This is a respiratory disease characterized by recurrent attacks of difficulty in breathing, usually accompanied by wheezing and coughing. It is due to an obstruction in the airway caused by a spasm of the muscle fibres in the walls of the bronchioles (the small air passages in the lungs). The spasm reduces the size of the airway and this restricts the flow of air. Asthma can occur at any age but is most common in children. It can occur anytime following birth but the higher incidence appears in children age 3 years and upwards. Childhood asthma sometimes disappears during the teenage years. Asthma does have an hereditary factor, often running in families, is more commonly found in males and it is not uncommon to find asthma sufferers also have eczema. In recent years there has been a marked increase in the incidence of childhood asthma although the reasons for this are unknown. Four main causes of asthma have been identified:

1. Direct irritation of the bronchiole membrane by dust, chemicals, air pollutants
2. Reflex irritation of the bronchiole membrane from infection elsewhere, i.e. sore throat, nasal infection, gastric infection
3. Allergy to pollen, animal fur, feather pillows, house dust, certain foods etc. In these cases the child may also suffer from eczema or other forms of dermatitis
4. Psychological factors such as fear, anxiety and severe emotional trauma may trigger an attack.

An acute asthma attack can be a very frightening thing for the child, parents or carer. The most important thing is to stay calm and reassure the child; if the child gets nervous or begins to panic it will make the attack far worse. If this is a first attack the doctor should be called immediately. It is important that the urgency of the situation is clearly relayed to the doctor. If the attack gets worse and the child is having great difficulty breathing and her colour is poor (blue around the lips and mouth, looks pale) then an ambulance should be sent for, ensuring that the emergency telephone operator is made aware that the patient is a child with serious breathing difficulties. An acute asthma attack will usually respond to the administration of drugs such as ephedrine, adrenaline, antihistamines etc.

Once the child has recovered from the acute attack phase the asthma is likely to be controlled with inhalers or other medicine. Doctors also may recommend a sensitivity test in order to try to determine whether the cause is an allergic reaction.

Coeliac Disease

This is an inherited (genetic) disease whereby the lining of the intestine is damaged by gluten, a protein found in wheat, rye, barley and some other cereals. The condition usually appears at the age of 6–24 months. The child will fail to thrive, will lose his appetite and have diarrhoea with bulky offensive stools. Diagnosis is made by taking a biopsy of a piece of the lining of the intestines. Once the diagnosis is made the disease is treated by giving a gluten free diet; this means eating only cereals where the gluten has been removed. Children with the condition will need to stay on this diet for the rest of their lives.

Conjunctivitis

This is an inflammation of the conjunctiva (membrane which covers the front of the eye). The eye may have a sticky discharge and the conjunctiva, which is normally colourless may appear pink; there may also be irritation as if a piece of grit had got into the eye. There are a number of bacteria and viruses which can cause conjunctivitis and it is also a complication of measles. It is easily remedied by getting prescription eye drops from the doctor. It is important to try to prevent the child rubbing the eye as the infection is easily spread to both eyes and to other children or family members.

Convulsions

A convulsion is a violent uncontrolled movement of muscles in the body which may be accompanied by loss of consciousness. A convulsion is always a serious sign and will always require medical attention. Febrile convulsions occur in some children when the child has a high temperature. They are most common in children aged from 1–3 years and usually do not occur in children over the age of 5 years. The doctor should be called immediately and whilst waiting for the doctor the parent or carer should try to bring the child's temperature down by tepid (not cold) sponging, cooling with an electric fan, opening windows, removing excessive clothing and bedcovers.

Cystic Fibrosis

This is an inherited (genetic) disease occurring in about one in 2000 births. Approximately one in 20 adults are carriers of the gene; where two carriers have a child there is a one in four chance of it having cystic fibrosis (this particular ratio is known as a Mendelian recessive). The gene is mainly found in people of Indo-European origin.

The condition affects all the mucus-secreting glands in the body whereby they do not secrete runny, watery discharge but thick viscous discharge which blocks the connecting tubes. It may be diagnosed in the first weeks of life due to failure to thrive, as the lack of pancreatic juices prevents the digestion of food; there is also diarrhoea with offensive faeces due to the inability to digest fat, and a cough due to chest infection. However, more commonly the diagnosis is made in the first few years of life with the child having repeated chest infections and the inability to digest foods. The diagnosis may be confirmed by examination of the child's faeces and its sweat, which will have a high sodium chloride (salt) content.

The long term management of the disease is by giving pancreatic enzymes, vitamin supplements and a low fat, high sodium chloride diet. Daily physiotherapy is carried out by the parents or carers in order to clear the mucus from the lungs.

Diabetes Mellitus

This is caused by the pancreas failing to secrete enough insulin, which prevents the body storing and using glucose. The glucose remains in the blood, and sugar is secreted in the urine. The incidence of diabetes in the population is increasing and is now at a level of about 1.5% of the population diagnosed as having the disease. Diabetes in the under-five age group is rare but one-fifth of all diagnosed diabetics are children. When young children develop diabetes there is usually a familial connection whereby another member of the family (possibly distant relative) has diabetes.

The first signs of diabetes are a sudden intense thirst accompanied by excessive urine output. If this stage goes undetected by parents or carers then the child is likely to become lethargic, drowsy and may go into a coma. It is easy to diagnose by urine and blood tests. Diabetes can be controlled by giving daily insulin injections in conjunction with a low carbohydrate diet. The amount of insulin given needs to be finely balanced as too much insulin can lead to the child going into a coma (hypoglycaemia) and too little can also lead to a coma (hyperglycaemia). Hypoglycaemia can happen very quickly and as it is the result of having too little sugar in the blood, sugar lumps or a high glucose drink will reverse the situation. Children often become familiar with the early warning signs of hypoglycaemia and should carry glucose tablets or sugar lumps in their pockets. If the child becomes unconscious before she can be given sugar/glucose then an ambulance must be called as she will require emergency treatment.

If the child has been eating foods which are not on her diet programme she may have too much sugar in her blood for the insulin to be able to neutralize; this will lead to a hyperglycaemic coma. The child must be seen immediately by a doctor and if the child is unconscious then an ambulance should be called. If the reason has been that the child has eaten too many sweets or other tempting goodies which she is not allowed, it is no use being cross with the child. It must be explained to the child that she does have an illness and how important it is for her to help control the illness by not eating forbidden foods. Although certain precautions need to be taken with diabetic children, they are usually able to lead a normal lifestyle, participating in all activities.

SCENARIO 2.2

Julia is a nanny caring for Jamie aged 18 months. Jamie has recently had a bad cold, with a raised temperature, and has been sleeping a lot. Julia goes to his bedroom to wake him after a nap and finds that he is twitching and writhing about in an uncontrolled fashion. What do you think is happening to Jamie? What action must Julia take?

Diarrhoea

This term refers to frequent bowel motions which pass loose, fluid faeces. For children the most dangerous side effect of diarrhoea is dehydration (sudden loss of fluid in the body) which can lead to death if it goes untreated. Diarrhoea in babies/young children is often accompanied by vomiting (gastroenteritis) and this is far more dangerous than diarrhoea alone. Babies who are bottle fed are very susceptible to gastroenteritis, which they can contract through infected feeding bottles. Bottle fed babies sometimes have diarrhoea due to too much sugar in the feed or the fat content of the milk being too high.

There are numerous causes of diarrhoea, such as infection, food poisoning, high temperature, or an allergy to cow's milk or a certain food. It can also be a symptom of another illness, e.g. coeliac disease or cystic fibrosis.

All cases of diarrhoea should be taken seriously, and if prolonged over a period of 24 hours in children over 2 years then medical advice should be sought. For children under 2 years medical advice should be sought at the onset. If it is accompanied by vomiting then medical advice should be sought immediately.

Eczema (Dermatitis)

Another name for eczema is dermatitis and both are generic terms for a number of different skin diseases. Eczema is an inflammation of the skin and is very common; one in eight children may suffer from this at some time in their lives. A common cause is thought to be external irritants which trigger the body's immune system to respond. Dermatologists are of the opinion that those people who suffer from eczema or other forms of dermatitis have a particularly sensitive immune system, and it is thought that the trait is inherited and is passed through families. It is not uncommon to find children who have eczema also suffering from more than one allergic illness, for example asthma or hayfever. Children may have a mild form of eczema or a severe form and it can last for a few months or over a number of years.

The doctor will be able to offer a number of remedies depending upon the type of rash and the severity of the rash (Box 2.2). It is also useful to try to avoid substances which may cause irritation to the skin, for example by using pure cotton garments next to the child's skin rather than wool or synthetic fibres. It is also better to use bath oils in place of soap and to use non-biological washing powders for the child's clothes. Putting cotton gloves on the child at night can prevent damage through scratching.

Box 2.2
*Characteristics of
eczema rash (Source:
The Great Ormond
Street Book of Baby
and Child Care by
Hilton T & Messenger
M published by
Bodley Head used by
permission of The
Random House
Group Limited.)*

Characteristic	Description
Itching	This is the worst aspect because it can be so upsetting for the child. It also makes them scratch, which can lead to more rawness, soreness and infection
Redness	This is caused by extra blood flowing through the blood vessels in the skin in the infected area
A bubbly, grainy appearance on the skin	These are tiny fluid-filled blisters just under the skin called 'vesicles'
Weeping	This happens when the blisters burst, either by themselves or because of scratching, and the fluid oozes out onto the surface of the skin
Crusts	These are scabs which form when the fluid dries
Scaliness	Children with eczema often have a dry, scaly skin. This may be a result of the disease but may also be the natural skin type of that family which, in some people, can predispose them towards developing eczema
Pigmentation	Pale patches of skin can appear because eczema can disturb the production of pigment which controls skin colour. The effect does fade and disappear
Lichenification	This means a leathery, thicker skin area in response to scratching. Again it does fade

Seborrhoeic dermatitis (cradle cap)

This type of dermatitis is not related to eczema or other types of dermatitis. Cradle cap occurs in young babies and is caused by the glands on the scalp producing too much sebum (grease). It appears as brown scaly patches which may cover the whole scalp. There is no need for medical treatment as the condition disappears of its own accord. Baby oil can be used to soften the crust. The health visitor will also be able to advise on the best type of shampoo to use when a baby has cradle cap.

Failure to Thrive (FTT)

This is not actually an illness but a cluster of symptoms which may be associated with some of the illnesses mentioned in this section. There appears to be no agreed definition of FTT but it is generally used to describe infants/children who fail to gain weight. It results from the failure to obtain or use the necessary calories required for growth. Betz et al (1994) describe three categories of FTT (see also Box 2.3):

1. *Organic FTT* is caused by physical factors such as congenital heart defects, gastrointestinal disorders, renal disease, central nervous system abnormalities, chronic infections, endocrine disorders.

2. *Non-Organic FTT* is an absence of any (medical) history, physical or laboratory findings that indicate organic disease capable of causing FTT. It is caused by environmental factors that affect the child's intake or use of calories. The problem is usually due to a complex set of interactive patterns between the infant and the care givers.

3. *Mixed FTT* is caused by a combination of organic and non-organic factors. For example, a child with a hare lip is unable to suck adequately because of the physical deformity (organic cause). The inability to suck, in turn, can interfere with the mother's feelings of adequacy. She may then stimulate and caress the infant less. The interplay of positive messages and reciprocal play associated with feeding is, therefore, blocked to a degree.

Box 2.3 *Indicators of potential failure to thrive*

Physical indicators
Weight below the 3rd percentile[1]
Sudden or rapid deceleration in the growth rate
Delay in developmental milestones
Muscular hypotonia (poor muscle tone)
Decreased muscle mass
Generalized weakness
Abdominal distension

Behavioural indicators
Avoiding eye contact
Intense watchfulness
Avoidance of physical contact with other people
Repetitive self-stimulating behaviours (e.g., rocking, head banging, head rolling, and intense sucking)
Disturbed affect (e.g. excessive irritability, apathy, or extreme compliance)
Sleep disturbances
Lack of age-appropriate stranger anxiety
Inappropriate lack of preference for parents

[1] Measurement relates to standard height/weight charts for normal development

There is a view that non-organic FTT is a symptom of child neglect caused by maternal deprivation. However, this is not the accepted view of all paediatricians as some advocate that whatever the cause it is a genuine clinical illness.

Glue ear

This is a very common condition affecting children under the age of 6 years. Modern hearing tests and diagnostic procedures have led to an increase in diagnosis of this condition. Glue ear is the name given to the condition whereby the fluid in the middle ear becomes viscous and glue-like, blocking the eustachian tube (the tube connecting the ear and the nose) and, if left untreated, is likely to damage a child's hearing. It is easily treated by inserting 'grommets' (tiny hollow tubes of plastic) into the ear drum to equalize the pressure within the ear drum and aid the draining of the fluid. 'Grommets' are inserted under a general anaesthetic so the child may have to stay in hospital overnight or attend a special day surgery unit at the hospital.

Haemophilia

This is a sex-linked inherited (genetic) disease which affects the clotting ability of blood. It affects males but is passed on through the female genes as the defect is on the sex-linked chromosome (there is a rare form of haemophilia which is not sex-linked and therefore affects both males and females and this is called Von Willebrand's disease). In haemophilia the blood is unable to clot due to a lack of the anti-haemophilic factor, commonly known as Factor 8. A child with haemophilia will get spontaneous bruising which is the result of bleeding into the skin tissues; there is also bleeding into the joints, such as knees, ankles and elbows, which make them appear red and swollen. Haemophiliac children need to be protected from boisterous play which may lead to injury or bleeding. Because of the spontaneous bruising, child care workers and health visitors may mistake an undiagnosed haemophiliac child as a victim of child abuse. It is therefore always wise to refer any cases of bruising in children to the paediatrician or GP to avoid misdiagnosis.

Haemophiliacs can be treated by transfusions of blood products which contain Factor 8. Sadly, some haemophiliacs were given Factor 8 from the USA which was contaminated with the HIV virus. From 1985 onwards all blood was carefully tested for HIV/AIDS and therefore this situation should not recur. Some of the haemophiliacs who were infected with the HIV virus have subsequently developed AIDS (Acquired Immune Deficiency Syndrome).

> **SCENARIO** 2.3
>
> You are in charge of a mixed age range group of children in a family centre. Beth aged 3 years is a new child and she is diagnosed as having cystic fibrosis. What information will you need to obtain from Beth's parents? Write a programme for Beth's daily routine. What, if any, special precautions will you need to take for Beth?

Headlice

Headlice are an infestation rather than an illness. They are parasites which live on hairs and feed by sucking the blood of the host. They are about 1–4 mm long, greyish white in colour and multiply at a very fast rate. They are very easily spread when children put their heads together or swop hats or hair ribbons etc. Headlice used to be viewed as a result of poor hygiene and children with headlice were stigmatized by being sent to special clinics; they were made to sit away from the other children and had to play alone. Fortunately, the progress of science has shown us how headlice are spread and how infestation is not necessarily associated with poor living conditions or neglect.

The first sign that a child may have headlice is that the parent or carer notices the child scratching its head due to irritation caused by the bites. A careful examination of the hair may reveal small white dots on the hairs, particularly behind the ears and at the nape of the neck. The white dots are the eggs of the lice (nits) which are fixed to the hair by a cement-like substance, so that unlike dandruff they do not flake off. The mature headlouse lays about 60 or more eggs a month and these take 7 days to hatch and are fully grown in about 2 weeks. Treatment is by the application of a special lotion which can be purchased from the chemist or obtained free from local health clinics. It is important to follow the instructions when applying the shampoo or lotion and the child's hair must be left to dry naturally as any applied heat, such as that from a hair dryer, will stop the chemicals taking effect. More recently the headlice have developed immunity to some of the special lotions and new ones are having to be developed. In order to try to counteract this happening, old fashioned methods are being turned to such as removing nits using vinegar and a special (sackers) comb.

If a child at nursery or school has become infested with headlice it is important that the staff take precautions to prevent the spread. All hats in the dressing-up corner should be removed and thoroughly washed in disinfectant. Each child should have their own comb and brush as a matter of routine good practice and these should be regularly washed and disinfected. Children's hats and coats should be kept on their own pegs and children should be discouraged from trying on each others hats, slides, ribbons etc. It is very important that the child is not ostracized or humiliated in front of the other children; the child is likely to be very frightened and will need a lot of reassurance and comforting.

Hepatitis

This is the name given to inflammation of the liver which in children is likely to be caused by a virus. There are two types of hepatitis virus, A and B. Most cases of hepatitis in the UK are caused by virus A, whereas hepatitis contracted abroad is most likely to be virus B. There are vaccinations against both types of hepatitis virus. Symptoms of hepatitis are loss of appetite, headache, fever and jaundice (where the skin and whites of the eyes become yellow). Hepatitis is very infectious and therefore strict hygiene precautions must be used when dealing with infected children. There is no specific treatment except rest and a high protein diet. Hepatitis is rare in young children.

HIV/AIDS

HIV (Human Immunodeficiency Virus) is the virus that is thought to cause AIDS (Acquired Immune Deficiency Syndrome), although not all HIV positive people develop AIDS. There is no test for AIDS; all that the scientists know at present is that people who have AIDS also test positive for HIV and that some people who are HIV positive have developed AIDS. The virus was first identified in the 1980s, although it is now known that there were cases of AIDS before this date but they went undiagnosed.

HIV is known to be transmitted in the following body fluids:

- Semen
- Vaginal and cervical secretions
- Blood
- Blood products, i.e. plasma, clotting factors.

Although HIV has been found in other body fluids such as saliva, urine, breast milk, tears and amniotic fluid, there is no evidence to show that it has ever been transmitted through these routes. The most common routes for transmission are through unprotected penetrative intercourse, and the sharing of syringes and needles by drug abusers.

There are three routes by which children may become infected with HIV:

1. Being a haemophiliac and becoming infected by being given infected blood products (see under haemophilia)

2. Having acquired the virus from their mothers
3. By being sexually abused by a person who is HIV positive. In these circumstances the transmission is the same as for the adult population.

Most of the children in the UK who are HIV positive have acquired it via their mothers, who are likely to have been drug abusers. Before birth the virus may be transmitted across the placenta to the developing fetus, during birth the virus may be transmitted via blood or vaginal and cervical secretions, and after birth it may possibly be transmitted in the breast milk.

Between 10% and 20% of HIV positive women will pass the virus to their baby. Doctors are unsure about breast milk being a route by which HIV is passed to children; however, HIV positive mothers are recommended not to breast feed their babies.

All babies whose mothers are HIV positive will have the mother's antibodies in their blood. These antibodies do not disappear until the child is around 2 years of age; it is therefore difficult to diagnose children under 2 years as definitively being HIV positive.

For the child care worker there is a greater risk of prejudice against children who are HIV positive than of them developing the disease; it is therefore important that the child care worker maintains a high level of confidentiality to avoid the child and family being stigmatized. As the Lambeth Women and Children's Health Project (1992) points out, 'There is no known case anywhere in the world of HIV infection having been transmitted in child care settings or schools.'

There are other infections such as hepatitis which are much more common than HIV and transmitted much more easily. There is therefore no reason why an HIV positive child should not be treated the same as all other children. Good hygiene practices should be followed at all times to protect workers and other children against infection (see Department of Health (1992) guidelines, pp. 37–40). It is very possible that a child care worker may not know which children are HIV positive; this will depend upon the confidentiality policy of the establishment or local authority. Under the Children Act 1989, HIV positive children come into the category of 'children in need' and this means that the local authority has a duty to ensure that help is provided for the families in order to enable them to meet the needs of the child.

Impetigo

This is a staphylococcal or streptococcal infection of the skin. It may develop as a complication of another skin complaint such as eczema or scabies. Impetigo starts with red spots which develop into blisters and these burst and form brownish crusts. It usually affects the scalp, face or hands. It is highly contagious (spread through touching) and extra care must be taken to prevent the spread of the infection to other children or carers. The doctor is able to prescribe antibiotics in the form of cream or tablets.

Nappy Rash

This is a rash that appears in the nappy area causing discomfort and pain for the baby. It can be caused by leaving the baby in a wet nappy and rubber pants for too long, as a reaction to detergents or biological soap powders, not properly drying the nappy area following a bath, or by the spread of seborrhoeic dermatitis from the baby's scalp (see under eczema).

It is treated by carefully cleaning the nappy area and then applying cream such as zinc and castor oil to the affected area to act as a waterproof barrier. The rash will heal more quickly if the baby can be left without a nappy for a few hours per day. Rubber pants should not be used and all nappies should be sterilized and washed in a detergent which is non-biological or specifically for baby clothes or children with allergies.

A more severe form of nappy rash can be caused by urine which is strong in ammonia. This type of rash is rarely seen in breast fed babies as the strong ammonia in the urine is caused by a bacteria which thrives in the conditions produced by cow's milk feeds.

SCENARIO 2.4

Jamila works in a playgroup as a volunteer. Jamila notices that a number of children in her group are frequently scratching their heads. What do you think is wrong with the children? What action will Jamila need to take? What should the playgroup leader tell the children's parents?

Rickets

This is a disease of the bones which is caused by lack of vitamin D. It used to be very common in the UK until the 1940s when the government started the fortification of margarine with vitamin D. With the introduction of better diets and free school milk the disease was virtually eradicated. However, the Rickets Report (Sheiham and Quick 1982) showed that there has been a significant increase in rickets and osteomalacia, particularly amongst Asian groups. Rickets is the name given to the disease when it occurs in children whose bones are still forming, and in adults it is called osteomalacia. Vitamin D is obtained from dietary sources or through the action of sunlight on the skin. Vitamin D is found in foods such as oily fish, liver, eggs etc. The prevalence of rickets and osteomalacia amongst the Asian community is mainly a result of their migration to the UK. People who have been used to living in the Asian sub-continent would have relied upon the sunshine to supply them with vitamin D and would not have needed to be concerned that they were getting this in their daily diet. However, following immi-gration to the UK they did not have the amount of sunshine they needed in order to keep up levels of vitamin D, and their diets may have changed very little from what they ate in Asia. Asians who have been born in the UK are likely to have a more varied dietary intake through school meals and eating in fast food establishments and restaurants; and through school nutrition projects and other health education programmes they are likely to be aware of the need for a diet rich in vitamin D. It is most likely that there is now less of an increase in rickets in the UK than there was in the 1980s, but there may still be an increase in osteomalacia amongst the older Asians.

Rickets leads to deformities of the bone such as bow legs or knock knees, and arm, skull and rib deformities. Osteomalacia leads to aching bones, listlessness and weakness of muscles in adults and fragile brittle bones in the elderly.

Ringworm (Tinea)

This is not a worm but a fungus which invades the skin, hair and nails. The fungus spreads down hair follicles and causes ring-shaped scaly patches. Ringworm is highly contagious and is easily spread to the other children or carers. It is easily treated with Griseofulvin ointment. Another type of infection caused by a similar fungus is athlete's foot which causes itching between the toes; this is most often transmitted in swimming baths and school shower rooms or other communal changing rooms.

Sickle Cell Disease

This is a term used to cover a number of blood diseases which are the result of an inherited (genetic) disorder of the haemoglobin in the red cells. The red blood cells become sickle shaped, hence the name of the illness. It is found in people who themselves or whose ancestors have come from African countries. Those with the sickle cell gene were protected from certain forms of malaria, thus it became a favoured gene in countries where there was malaria. In the UK the gene is carried by Africans, Afro-Caribbeans, people from the Middle East, South Asia and the Mediterranean. Mares et al (1985) estimated that one in 400 of the UK's African and Afro-Caribbean population had sickle cell disease and one in 10 were carriers of the gene. In order for a child to inherit the disease they must have two parents who have the gene. With both parents carrying the gene the child will have a one in four chance of inheriting the disease. If only one parent has the gene then the child will have a 50/50 chance of being a carrier of the disease. Carriers of the disease are described as having sickle cell trait.

The first symptoms of sickle cell do not usually appear until the child is 3–6 years of age. The sickle shaped cells only live for 10–20 days, unlike normal red blood cells which live for approximately 120 days. The constant breakdown of the sickle cells causes chronic anaemia. The shape of the cells makes it difficult for them to pass along small blood vessels and they can become clumped together and stop the blood supply; this often occurs in the hands and feet. When this happens the child will have a lot of pain and this is described as a sickle cell crisis. A crisis can also be brought on by dehydration, strenuous exercise and infection. The constant breaking down of the red cells also leads to enlargement of the spleen. Sickle cell is diagnosed by a blood test. There is no routine screening in the UK for those children who are thought to be at risk from the disease, unlike the USA where a 1972 Act of Congress ensures that there are services for voluntary screening and diagnosis, counselling, education, medical referral and research. Sickle cell disease is not always easy to diagnose as the symptoms may be slight and may only be discovered during a routine blood test before an anaesthetic or during pregnancy.

There is no cure for sickle cell disease and the treatment is one that aims to relieve the symptoms. There is a good prognosis for sickle cell sufferers, and as medical science makes progress so they are able to have a longer and longer life span.

Parents and carers of a child with sickle cell disease will need clear and practical information on how to manage the child's condition. There is a Sickle Cell Society (details can be found in the Appendix at the back of this book) which is able to offer information and support to sufferers, families and those who are working with people that have the disease. As with any genetic disease, parents will often feel very guilty, as they are responsible for their child's condition. It is therefore important that child care workers appreciate this and treat the parents with a high level of understanding and sensitivity.

Thalassaemia

Like sickle cell disease, thalassaemia is an inherited (genetic) blood disorder. It mainly occurs in people from the Mediterranean areas such as Spain, Cyprus, Portugal, Italy etc., but there are also people with this gene who come from North Africa and India. It is inherited in the same ratios as sickle cell disease; those with the disease are described as having thalassaemia major and those who are carriers are described as having thalassaemia minor.

In thalassaemia the red blood cells are unable to produce haemoglobin which operates efficiently, as it is unable to utilize iron. It can be diagnosed during the first 6 months of life as these children have severe anaemia and show symptoms of failing to thrive. It is treated by giving blood transfusions, and bone marrow transplants have proved successful. Sufferers also need regular injections of a drug which will counteract the excessive amounts of iron in their bloodstream. There is a good prognosis for thalassaemia sufferers, although there is no cure for the condition. It is possible, in rare cases, for children to have both sickle cell anaemia and thalassaemia.

REST AND SLEEP

In order for children to stay healthy they need an adequate amount of rest and sleep. Sleep enhances tissue restoration and enables the body to relax, which promotes alertness during the waking hours. Children who are tired are more susceptible to infections and tend to be bad tempered and fretful. New babies will soon establish a pattern between waking and sleeping which is usually associated with feeding times. As they get older they will sleep for fewer hours but no two children are alike in their sleep patterns and some children may need less sleep than others. Children, like adults, will develop their own individual sleep patterns. Adults need to encourage children from an early age to develop different sleeping patterns for night and day. This can be done by giving the baby a great deal of stimulation during its daytime waking periods and trying not to give any stimulation during night-time waking periods. Giving the baby a bath before putting it down to sleep will relax it and prepare it for bed.

Although children need a comfortable place to sleep, this does not necessarily mean their own bed; sleeping arrangements will differ between families and cultures. In some cultures it is traditional for small children, even babies, to sleep in the same bed as their parents. There used to be a fear that taking a baby into bed with adults put it at risk of being suffocated by the adult rolling on top of the baby. Dr Hugh Jolly (1985) points out that slow motion films of babies in bed with their parents have shown that a normal baby will wriggle its way into a position so that it can breathe easily and that parents have a tendency to roll away from the baby. The only rider to this is that the adults must not be under the influence of alcohol or sleeping pills, as this dulls their normal reactions which would safeguard the baby. In the UK it is common practice that most children have their own cot/bed which is surrounded by their favourite toys, although this may be in the bedroom of the parents or the room of a sibling.

Most parents look forward to the day when their baby will sleep throughout the night; however some children may do this at an early age, whereas others might take longer. It is important to develop a bedtime routine with children. This usually starts with bath time, saying goodnight to the family and being read a story once they are tucked up in bed with their favourite toy.

As they increase their waking hours, most children will need a nap during the day. In the early days this will be mid-morning and another mid-afternoon. Once children are old enough to go to playgroup or part-time nursery school, it is easier if they have their nap during the part of the day that they are at home. Most playgroups and nursery schools do not have facilities for children to have a nap. If a child is in a day care situation then the child care worker will need to talk to the parent about the child's sleeping habits. She will need to find out when the child likes to go to sleep, what favourite toy or comforter he likes to have with him when he sleeps, whether he has a story before sleeping and how long he is likely to sleep for.

As children get older and become interested in television, it becomes more difficult to get them to bed at a reasonable time. Parents and carers must be firm about keeping to a specific bedtime as children who are tired during the day have difficulty concentrating and this inhibits their learning.

As children get older they may develop fears which either prevent them from sleeping or make them wake up during sleep. Children, like adults, will have dreams and nightmares, but they are too young to recognize these and talk about them. It is a good idea to leave a small electric night-light on in the child's room so that if he does wake he does not find himself in complete darkness. Children who are frightened to go to sleep may be worried that their carer is going to leave them, so it always a good idea to put them to bed yourself and to reassure them that if they wake up you will be there.

EXERCISE

All children need exercise, room to move around and stretch their limbs, and time in the open air. Movement and exercise help children's physical development and give them the opportunity to develop muscle coordination and gross motor movements. A period of time in the open air will stimulate the circulation of the blood, enable them to obtain vitamin D from the sunshine and improve their appetite. Recent research has shown that children in the UK are becoming overweight due to poor diet and lack of exercise. Most children are able to gain enough exercise by being given regular opportunities to play indoors and outdoors. Outings are an important activity for children. Visits to the local playground, the zoo, inner city farm or just the local park are able to offer children an exciting experience as well as exercise. Many children live in cramped conditions or high rise flats and do not get the opportunity to play outside; the nursery or playgroup is able to offer them this on a regular daily basis. As long as children are dressed appropriately there is no need for the weather to prevent them playing outdoors. This is well proven in Denmark where there is a form of pre-school provision called 'forest kindergarten'. Children are collected from the city and taken by bus to a wooded area where they spend the whole day outdoors.

ASSIGNMENTS

1. Write an essay on why it is important for the child care worker to have good personal hygiene habits.

2. Write an essay debating the advantages and disadvantages of immunizing children against whooping cough (pertussis).

3. Describe the special care that you would need to give to a 6-year-old child in your class who has been diagnosed as having sickle cell disease.

4. Write an account of how you would deal with a 4-year-old child who is having an asthma attack.

5. What do you understand by the term 'health screening'? Write an essay explaining what this is and its relevance to child health.

PRACTICAL ACTIVITIES

1. Visit your local infant welfare clinic or GP surgery and write a comprehensive account of what the clinic/surgery is able to offer parents and young children.

2. Produce a leaflet for parents on the problem of headlice, stating how these are spread and how they can be treated.

3. Carry out an audit in your work setting or placement to find where policies on dealing with sick children are kept and the named people responsible.

4. Draw up a weekly menu for a child suffering from coeliac disease.

5. Undertake a survey in your work setting or placement of those children who need a nap during the day. Represent your findings by drawing a graph showing children's ages on one axis and length of time sleeping on the other axis.

References

Betz CL, Hunsberger M, Wright S 1994 Family-centred nursing care of children, 2nd edn. WB Saunders, Philadelphia

Department of Health 1992 Children and HIV: guidance for local authorities. HMSO, London

Hilton T, Messenger M 1993 The Great Ormond Street book of baby and child care. Bodley Head, London

Jolly H 1985 Book of child care. Unwin, London

Lambeth Women and Children's Health Project 1992 HIV/AIDS: A guide for carers of young children. Lambeth Women and Children's Health Project, London

Mares P, Henley A, Baxter C 1985 Health care in multi-racial Britain. Health Education Council and National Extension College, Cambridge

Sheiham H, Quick A 1982 The Rickets Report. Haringey Community Health Council, London

Further reading

- Claxton R, Harrison T 1991 Caring for children with HIV and AIDS. Edward Arnold, London

- Department of Health and Social Security 1980 Rickets and osteomalacia. Report of the working party on fortification of food with vitamin D. Committee on medical aspects of food policy. HMSO, London

- Griffiths R (ed) 1992 HIV/AIDS and the under fives. A guide for workers and carers. Manchester AIDSline Women's Group, Manchester

- Leach P 1989 Baby and child: from birth to age five. Penguin, London

- Leach P 1997 Your baby and child. Penguin, London

- O'Hagan M, Smith M 1999 Early years childcare and education: key issues. Baillière Tindall, London

- VOLCUF 1991 Keeping children healthy – a guide for under fives workers. VOLCUF, London

Chapter 3

Child Safety

This chapter covers underpinning knowledge for all or parts of the following unit from the National Vocational Qualifications (NVQs) in Child Care and Education: E2. It is also linked to the following CACHE awards Units: Diploma Units 3, 9; Certificate Unit 1.

INTRODUCTION

It is a major responsibility of all child care workers to ensure that children are always in an environment which is safe. Accidents are the highest cause of deaths in children aged between 1–14 years. For children under the age of 5 years it is mostly accidents within the home which are responsible for the highest numbers of deaths. Under the registration procedures for the Children Act 1989 all premises where children are cared for must reach minimal levels of safety. It is the responsibility of the carer to ensure that these levels of safety are maintained from day to day and that they do not deteriorate following the visit of the registration officer. All child care workers should be familiar with the safety regulations of their setting, for example what to do in the event of a fire or the need to evacuate the nursery or playgroup. Child care workers also need to know who is responsible for health and safety in the setting and the policies relating to the safety of toys and equipment, the outdoor area etc.

A number of child care workers are nannies working in private houses who are not required to be registered under the Children Act 1989. For these people there is a responsibility to ensure that their employers are made aware of any areas in the house that may be unsafe and how these can be altered to make a child-safe environment.

Chapter 2 deals with safety in relation to infection and hygiene and this chapter concentrates on safety in the environment and protecting children. Child care workers will feel more confident to cope in the event of an accident if they hold a First Aid Certificate which is regularly updated.

FACTORS CONTRIBUTING TO ACCIDENTS

There are a number of factors that can contribute to accidents; these can be divided into human factors and environmental factors.

Human Factors

- Ignorance on the part of the carer about safety regulations. Ignorance is not a defence in a court of law; the person would still be held responsible as he has a duty to familiarize himself with safety regulations
- Carelessness and lack of observation on the part of the carer. This may be due to tiredness or fatigue or the carer having other things on his mind at the time
- Illness of the carer, which may affect his alertness to risky situations
- Influence of drugs or alcohol on the carer, which may make him careless or unaware of what is happening around him
- Not carrying out the routine safety procedures which have been explained to him or that he knows that he should be observing.

No carers should be left in sole charge of more children than they can be reasonably expected to control or keep safe. The Children Act guidelines clearly state the ratio of adults to children in a variety of settings and these should be adhered to at all times. It is particularly important when a carer is taking children off the premises on a visit or outing.

Environmental Factors

- The siting of buildings and outdoor play areas can increase the risk of accidents
- Lack of gates or doors to prevent children wandering out of the room or building
- The internal arrangements in the home or nursery, particularly in relation to safety in kitchens, bathrooms, toilets and stairs
- Safety of furniture, play equipment, heaters, bedding, cots and windows
- Safe storage of sharp implements such as knives, scissors, cooking equipment
- Safety of clothing and footwear, particularly fire-retardant nightwear.

The following are just some of the ways in which child care workers can make the environment safe for children in their care. The Child Accident Prevention Trust and the Royal Society for the Prevention of Accidents (addresses in Appendix) are able to provide very full explanatory leaflets on safety. Equipment bought for the home should have a British Standards Institute (BSI) Kite Mark if it is a cooker or other large piece of household equipment. Toys should have the lion mark to show that they have met British safety standards. The CE mark on equipment means that it complies with

British and European safety standards. Unfortunately there is not enough space in this book to go into full details on accident prevention and the following represent just some of the precautions that can be taken.

ACCIDENT PREVENTION IN THE HOME

The Kitchen

All sharp implements should be kept in drawers or cupboards that have childproof fastenings (these are readily available in most DIY stores). All cookers should have a safety guard on the top to prevent children reaching up and pulling over saucepans (available from stores such as Boots, Mothercare and DIY stores). When the cooker is in use, all pan handles should be turned towards the back of the cooker so that they do not jut out across the top of the stove. Kitchens should be equipped with a fire extinguisher and/or fire blanket. Children should not be left alone in the kitchen. The doorway to the kitchen should have a gate to prevent children entering. All detergents, cleaning fluids etc. should be kept in a cupboard high enough to be beyond the reach of children. If such items are kept under the sink unit then the doors should have childproof latches. Fridges and freezers should have locks that need a key in order to open them. Tables should not have cloths as a child can topple a pot of tea or other hot drink by pulling the cloth. All electrical plugs should be of the safety childproof type. Electrical points should have safety covers on when not in use in order to prevent children poking things into them. Any doors leading to the garden should have safety gates for use when the door may be left open, e.g. in the summer months.

The Lounge/ Sitting Room

All furniture should be stable and not tip easily when a child leans on it. All electrical plugs should be of the child safety type to prevent children poking objects into the empty sockets. Coffee tables should be stable and should not have glass surfaces. Any ornaments or other precious artefacts should be kept on high shelves well away from the reach of children. Television sets, video machines and hi-fi equipment should be placed well out of reach of the children, as should tapes, CDs and records. Video machines can now be purchased with a child lock in order to prevent children using adult or other unsuitable videos. Carpets should have non-slip surfaces and rugs should be backed with a non-slip substance. All fires or other exposed heating equipment should have a guard that is fixed to the wall. Windows should have child safety locks and bottom windows should not be opened when children are around, even in rooms on the ground floor. It is possible to get special safety devices which prevent windows being opened to a height which would enable a child to get through; these are available from good quality builders' merchants or DIY stores. There should be no trailing flexes or other objects that could cause a child to fall. If furniture has rough corners these should have protectors, which can be obtained from children's equipment shops such as Boots or Mothercare.

The Bathroom/ Toilet

All medicine cupboards should be situated well out of the reach of the child and medicines should be in a cupboard which has a lock. Cleaning fluids should be kept in a locked cupboard or on a shelf which children cannot reach from the floor height or when they may stand on the toilet cover. When bathing children the cold water must always be put in before the hot water. The hot water temperature should be turned down so that it is not of a heat that would scald a small child were she to turn on the hot tap. The bath must always be emptied before leaving the bathroom as the child may come along later and fall into the water. Electrical equipment such as hair dryers should not be left in bathrooms. Bathrooms should not have open socket plugs but closed sealed electrical systems for heaters, razors points etc. (this applies as a general safety rule even when there are no children in the household). If the bathroom door has a lock this should be of the type that can be opened from the outside in the event of a child accidentally locking herself in.

The Bedroom

All bedding, pillows and mattresses should conform to the safety regulations for children's bedding. If they are purchased from a reputable shop they will be clearly marked with one of the recognized safety kitemarks. Cots must have bars that are close enough together to prevent the child's head being able to get through them and they must be painted with non-toxic paint. All toys should have the lion safety kitemark, particularly if they have eyes that might come loose. All children's nightwear should be fire retardant. Any open fires should be guarded with a fixed fireguard. Any windows should have safety locks and should only open at the top. Any furniture should be low enough to prevent children climbing up to the height of the window. All electrical plugs should be child safe and there should be no exposed or trailing wires.

The Garden

All gardening tools should be kept away from children, preferably in a locked garden shed. Any ponds or pools should be covered with strong wire to prevent children falling into them. Swimming pools should have special covers that can be purchased from pool suppliers.

SCENARIO 3.1

Angela is a nanny who cares for Simon who is 18 months and Vanessa who is 3 years. Angela is visiting another nanny, Monica, who cares for Sarah aged 2 years. The children are playing in the sitting room with Angela and Monica. Suddenly Angela smells burning. What action should Angela and Monica take?

A special play area should be set aside for children where a swing or slide or other permanent fixed outdoor toy can be placed. It is best to fix such equipment in a grassed area so that if a child falls it is onto a soft surface rather than hard e.g. concrete. Alternatively there are special rubber or woodchip surfaces which can be purchased specifically to act as a surface for outdoor equipment. Any plants which may be toxic to children (e.g. foxgloves, nightshade), should be removed from the garden. All weedkillers, fertilizers and other garden chemicals should be kept locked in the garden shed.

KEEPING BABIES SAFE

Babies are very vulnerable and will need special precautions for their safety during the first months of life. Babies need a safe place to sleep which:

- Is free of pillows, which can easily suffocate a baby
- Does not have fluffy blankets, particles of which can get into a baby's mouth and cause choking
- Is stable and not able to be tipped over if the baby moves around
- Does not have hanging mobiles that the baby can reach
- Does not contain toys with small parts that a baby could swallow
- Has high enough sides to prevent the baby rolling out of the bed.

Babies are born with a very strong natural grasping reflex and they can quite easily pull pieces of material or other objects from toys or bedding. Avoid dressing children in lacy knitwear or clothing in which they can catch their fingers; ribbons around the neck can lead to choking.

A baby must not be left with a bottle propped in its mouth as this can lead to choking.

To help reduce the risk of cot death the Department of Health (1991) issued the following guidance:

- Lay babies on their backs to sleep
- Do not overwrap or overheat them
- Do not expose them to cigarette smoke.

> **SCENARIO** 3.2
>
> You have been asked to move into a friend's house for 3 weeks in order to dog-sit whilst she is on holiday. You will be taking your 18-month-old daughter with you. Before moving into the house you make a visit to check that it is safe for your daughter. What will you be looking for? Describe what you will need to do in order to make this a safe environment for your daughter.

Always keep small objects out of a baby's reach and if you leave the baby alone make sure the environment is safe. Always ensure that the baby has good support for head and back. At bath time put the cold water in the bath first and test the temperature before putting the baby into the water. Never leave a baby alone on a changing table.

SAFETY WHEN TAKING CHILDREN ON OUTINGS OR OUTSIDE THE HOME

Children should always be strapped securely into prams, pushchairs or buggies. When children begin to walk they should be kept on reins. If older children have a tendency to wander away from the carer, there is a restraining rein that can be purchased. The restraining rein is able to give the child a certain amount of freedom whilst at the same time ensuring that there is a link with the carer.

Children should be suitably dressed for the outing in clothes which protect them against the weather, hot, cold, wet or damp. Children should not wear their 'best' clothes and parents should be encouraged to dress them in casual clothes that do not require special cleaning or laundering. Children's clothing needs to allow them freedom of movement so that they can take full advantage of all the opportunities offered on the outing.

As soon as children are walking they should be introduced to road safety. At an early age, this is done by the example of the carer. Always cross roads at safe points such as traffic lights, zebra or pelican crossings. Always stop with the child at the kerb and check the flow of traffic. Never take a child across a road when it is unsafe, e.g. when traffic lights are on amber, when you can see a car approaching but may think it is going slowly, or from the side of parked vehicles which may restrict a driver seeing you. If children are exposed to consistently good examples of how to behave when crossing the road they will find it easier when they are older and have to learn to cross roads by themselves.

When taking children on an outing it is important that this is properly organized, whether it is a day out from the nursery or a

small group of children going to the local shop to buy cooking ingredients or pet food. Always check the nursery policy on taking children off the premises before embarking on any outing. In most establishments it requires parental permission in order to take a child off the premises. In some cases, members of staff may also need the permission of their line manager in order to take children off the premises.

There must always be a sufficient number of adults to cope with the number of children going out, and the minimum ratio for this can be obtained from the local authority registration officer and should be written down as part of the nursery or playgroup policy. In many instances parents may agree to accompany a group on an outing and this will increase the number of adults available to help. All outings should be planned in advance and parents and carers given full details in a letter about what is happening, when it is going to happen, length of the visit/outing and an invitation for them to join the outing. The bottom section of the letter can be a returnable permission slip which parents/carers need to sign.

Any outing with children needs to be well planned. It is always a good idea to visit the place you are going to in advance so that you can be sure of the facilities that are available and the areas that may be a danger to children, and can identify suitable places that can be used as meeting points if the party becomes separated.

It is very important that the organizer of the outing has a full list of all the children who are going on the outing. It is also a good idea to make name badges for all the children. Trying to cope with a very large group can be difficult; it is much easier to split the children into smaller groups and give the adults a specific group to be responsible for. The person in charge of the outing needs to be sure that all necessary equipment is ready before the day of the outing and to decide who will be responsible for this on the day. Items such as tissues, spare clothing, sports equipment, small first aid kit etc. are the type of things that may be needed.

Transportation may be booked in advance, e.g. minibus, coach or public transport. If private cars are being used the children should travel in the back seats and be secured by seat belts or special child seats. Car doors should have childproof locks. The use of private cars requires the owner/driver to ensure that his insurance company will give him cover if he transports children from his workplace in his car. If public transport is to be used the organizer should undertake a 'dummy run' in advance in order to identify any potential hazards or parts of the journey that may be difficult. It is essential that the person leading the party knows exactly where he is going and how he is going to get there. It is sensible to write this down for all the accompanying staff and helpers so that in the event of the party being separated, all those involved will know how to reach the final destination.

EMERGENCY SITUATIONS

Every carer hopes that she will never be in the situation of having to face an emergency but it is her duty, as a responsible person, to ensure that she would know what to do should such a situation arise. The most important thing in an emergency is to stay calm and not panic. The worker's first duty is to the children in her care, not her own safety, although it must be remembered that she will be no use to the children if she puts her own safety in jeopardy by trying to take unnecessary heroic action.

It is essential that the person looking after the child has up-to-date and accurate records of how to contact the child's parents or carer. This applies to all child care workers, even nannies, who must have the workplace contact number for at least one of the parents or carers.

All child care establishments should have regular fire drills, and all staff should know how to evacuate the children quickly and safely in the event of an emergency. The action to take in the event of a fire should be clearly displayed in the nursery or playgroup, and all staff should make themselves familiar with these instructions. Staff should also know the position of fire extinguishers and know where special extinguishers are located e.g. those for electrical fires. Exits which are designated as fire exits should be clearly marked and must never be blocked by equipment or furniture.

All child care establishments and childminders should maintain an accident book. Any injuries or accidents, however minor, to staff or children are recorded in this book. In each establishment there will be a specific person who is responsible for keeping the accident book. Records of accidents should contain the date and time that the accident happened, the name of the child/staff member who had the accident, which staff member was present at the time of the accident, what type of accident occurred, what the injuries were and who gave first aid. It is useful for all child care workers to have taken a first aid course. These may be organized by the St. John's Ambulance Service or the British Red Cross, or a local college may run its own short course. All establishments should have a named first-aider who has gained a diploma in dealing with accidents at work. Most of the first aid awarding bodies require their diplomas to be updated every 3–5 years.

Whenever children have an accident it is important to comfort and reassure them, however minor the injury may seem. All accidents must be reported to parents or carers. In the event of a serious accident occurring, the child care worker should inform whoever is in charge of the nursery or playgroup and this responsible person will then call a doctor or ambulance and inform the parents. Where the child care worker is in sole charge then he will be responsible for deciding on the seriousness of the injury, calling a doctor or ambulance and informing the parents or carer.

SCENARIO 3.3

Julia is a childminder caring for Sean aged 3 years and Sophie aged 1 year. Julia has teenage sons, Rory and Malcolm. The children are with Rory and Malcolm in the sitting room watching TV whilst Julia is in the kitchen preparing tea. Rory puts his cup of hot tea on the coffee table and he does not notice Sophie crawling nearby. Before Rory realizes it, Sophie has pulled the cup of hot tea over herself and is screaming. What action must Julia and Rory take to deal with this emergency?

DEALING WITH STRANGERS

As children get older (3–8 years) they will need to be alerted to other dangers which are outside the home. Unfortunately we do not live in a safe society; not all adults that children encounter will have the child's safety at heart. It is important that children are made aware of these dangers without alarming the children or making them frightened when they meet any new adult. Leach (1997) points out that it is not always useful to tell children not to talk to strangers when we are not able to identify for them who these strangers are. It is very difficult to describe to a child exactly who counts as a friend and who counts as a stranger. Leach advocates that it is better to tell children never to go anywhere with anybody without telling their parent or carer where they are going. This takes the decision out of the child's hands and also ensures that the child feels secure in knowing where its parent or carer is. This advice seems very sensible and can be started at an early age. As children get older they do want more freedom, but this must be balanced with ensuring that children are kept safe. Unfortunately, it is frequently the case that those people who do abuse children are not strangers to the child or the family. Many schools and playgroups use organizations such as Kidscape (address in Appendix) to teach children how to keep themselves safe. Kidscape will send a specially trained worker to carry out training sessions with the children. Kidscape training sessions are based upon helping children to be more assertive when they are in situations that make them feel uncomfortable. All child care establishments should have a policy regarding the collection of children. Children should not be allowed to leave the premises with a person who is unauthorized to collect them. If the parent/carer has made arrangements for a different person to collect the child then the establishment must be told in advance.

KEEPING CHILDREN SAFE FROM ABUSE

Child abuse has always been present in our society but it has not always been defined or recognized as damaging to the child. The first physical child abuse case was brought before a USA court in 1857 (Allen and Morton 1961) and had to be brought under laws pertaining to the cruelty of animals as there were no laws relating to the abuse of children. This famous case led to the founding of the National Society for the Prevention of Cruelty to Children (NSPCC) and the first laws to protect children from physical abuse were passed in 1889.

In 1968 Professor Kempe (Kempe & Kempe 1978), an American paediatrician, put forward the idea of the 'battered child syndrome' and he stated that there were four factors present in child abuse cases:

1. The parents must have a background of emotional or physical deprivation and perhaps abuse as well
2. A child must be seen as unlovable or disappointing
3. There must be a crisis
4. There are no effective sources of aid at the moment of crisis.

Research since the 1960s has shown that child abuse is a far more complex matter than the four factors offered by Kempe.

As society has come to learn more about child abuse it has become easier for those working with children to recognize the signs and obtain help for the family. Statistics are now kept, and with these and the high profile that the media has given to serious abuse cases, it would appear to be a prevalent problem within our society. It is difficult to prove that child abuse was common in the past as there are no statistics or records; however, some forms of child abuse are well documented in fictional works by people such as Dickens and in the work that Shaftesbury and Barnardo were doing.

There are a number of definitions of the different types of child abuse and each local authority will have these listed in their child protection documentation. The Open University uses the NSPCC definitions with some enhancements to include examples, as follows:

Neglect Where parents (or whoever else is caring for the child) fail to meet the basic essential needs of children, like adequate food, clothes, warmth and medical care. Leaving young children alone and unsupervised is another example of neglect; refusing or failing to give adequate love and affection is a case of emotional neglect.

Physical Abuse Where a parent (or somebody else caring for the child) physically hurts, injures or kills a child. This can involve hitting, shaking, squeezing, burning and biting. It also involves giving a child poisonous substances, inappropriate drugs and alcohol and attempted suffocation and drowning. It includes the excessive use of force when carrying out tasks like feeding or nappy changing.

Sexual Abuse When adults seek sexual gratification by using children (boys or girls). This may be by having sexual intercourse or anal intercourse (buggery), engaging with the child in fondling, masturbation or oral sex; and includes encouraging children to watch sexually explicit behaviour or pornographic material, including videos.

Emotional Abuse Where children are harmed by constant lack of love and affection, or threats, verbal attacks, taunting or shouting.

(Open University 1989)

In addition to the above definition the Department of Health defines one more category:

Grave Concern This category should not be used lightly and should be needed only in exceptional circumstances for children whose situations do not currently fit the above categories. This may be where there is an explicit and serious concern that the child is not developing as would be expected (and all medical causes have been eliminated) or there is sudden, unexplained change in that child's normal behaviour pattern. If the cause of the child's condition is later established as fitting one of the above categories, a case conference should amend the cause of registration.

(Department of Health 1991)

Indicators of Physical Abuse

- Unexplained bruising in places where an injury cannot easily be sustained or explained
- Facial bruising
- Hand or finger marks or pressure bruising
- Bite marks
- Burns (particularly cigarette burns), scalds
- Unexplained fractures
- Lacerations or abrasions.

Behavioural Indicators of Physical Abuse

- Shying away from physical contact
- Withdrawn or aggressive behaviour
- Sudden changes in behaviour, e.g. from extrovert to introvert.

Indicators of Sexual Abuse

- Bruises or scratches inconsistent with accidental injury
- Difficulty in walking or sitting
- Pain or itching in the genital area
- Torn, stained or bloody underclothes
- Bedwetting, sleep disturbances
- Loss of appetite.

Sites of injury to children: accidental and non-accidental

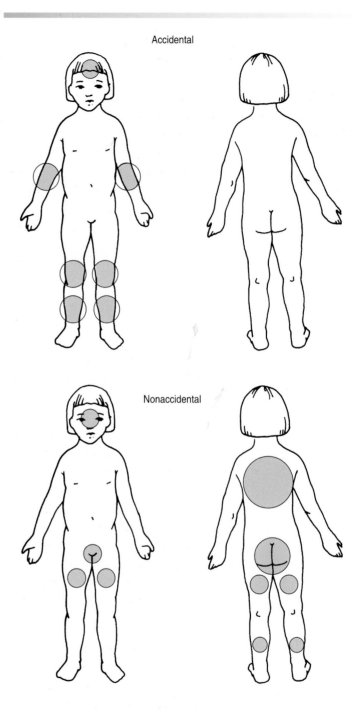

Accidental

Nonaccidental

Behavioural Indicators of Sexual Abuse

- Hints of sexual activity through words, play, drawings etc.
- Sexually precocious, uses seductive behaviour towards adults
- Uses sexually explicit language
- Excessive preoccupation with sexual matters
- Informed knowledge of adult sexual behaviour

- Poor self-esteem
- Withdrawn or isolated from other children.

ROLE OF THE CARER IN CHILD PROTECTION

Child care workers are not child protection experts or child psychologists and should not attempt to take on these roles. Child care workers are able to help children by listening to them, observing them and reporting their findings to the appropriate person so that the child can get the help that it needs. Children who have suffered abuse are vulnerable and this must be remembered when carers deal with these children.

The child care worker may or may not know which children in his care are designated as 'at risk' from abuse. If a child care worker does have information about a child's 'at risk' status then he must maintain strict confidentiality on this matter at all times. It is not always easy to spot signs of child abuse and for the carer the most indicative sign that something is wrong with a child is a change in the child's behaviour. However, the carer must beware of jumping to conclusions, as child abuse is not the only reason for a change in a child's behaviour. A major role of the child care worker is to observe the children in his care and report anything which may give him cause for concern. It is a good idea to observe a child on a number of occasions during the day and write down these observations. At the end of the day these observations can be discussed with the carer's immediate superior or co-worker.

If a carer finds bruising or other physical signs on a child during the routine process of changing a child's clothes then he must report this immediately to his superior. All carers should be aware of the local authority child protection policy. If a child discloses information to its carer this must be treated with sensitivity. At no time should the worker tell the child that he does not believe her. As the Department of Health document *Working Together* (1991) states:

> A child's statement about an allegation of abuse, whether in confirmation or denial, should always be taken seriously. A child's testimony should not be regarded as inherently less reliable than that of an adult. However, professionals need to be aware that a false allegation may be a sign of a disturbed family environment and an indication that the child may need help.

The carer should tell the child that he believes her and that he is glad that she has told him. The carer should also express sympathy and sadness that it has happened to the child. The child may feel that it is her fault and will therefore need reassurance. Carers are there to listen to the child and report what they have heard; they must not press children for details or question them. The carer should also tell the child that he will do his best to protect her and help her in the future.

In more recent years we have seen a number of situations where child care workers have abused children in their care. It is the duty of all child care workers to protect the children in their care and if they see fellow workers abusing children then they must report this to their superiors. If it is the superiors who are involved in the abuse then the child care worker must report the incidents to the local social services department. However, before doing any of the above child care workers must be very certain of their evidence and should keep clear and accurate records of what they have observed.

There are other things that happen in the child care situation which may not be viewed as abuse but which hurt children emotionally and physically, such as withholding food, making children eat food they do not like, humiliating children in front of other children and workers (using punishments such as 'naughty chairs'), threatening children verbally ('If you do not sit down I will telephone your mother') etc. All of these things hurt children emotionally and lead them to have low self-esteem. Such methods must not be used to control children.

ASSIGNMENTS

1. Plan an outing for a small group of 3 year olds. The plan should include all the preparations that need to be made in advance and on the day.

2. Describe accurately, including diagrams and room layouts, the procedures you would take when you hear the fire alarm in your workplace.

3. You are supervising outdoor play when Gemma, aged 3 years, falls down the steps on the slide. What immediate action do you take? What follow-up action may be required?

4. Describe how you would teach a small group of 4 year olds about road safety.

5. Describe the role of the child care worker in relation to child protection.

PRACTICAL ACTIVITIES

1. Collect copies of the establishment's Health and Safety Policy, Child Protection Policy and policies on taking children on outings. Put these in a file and keep a log of how often you need to refer to them.

2. Undertake a safety audit of the outdoor play area in the setting where you work.

3. Make a poster for older children (3–5 year olds or 5–7 year olds) which introduces them to the Green Cross Code. Follow this up by taking a short session with the children in which you tell them about the poster.

4. Visit your local supplier of children's toys and make a list of those toys which carry the lion mark. Note any other kite marks that you might find and check with the store as to what these mean.

5. With the permission of your superior/s, undertake an audit of the establishment's accident book and identify the most common accidents that have been reported during the past year. Discuss your results with your superior/s.

References

Allen A, Morton A 1961 This is your child: the story of the National Society for Prevention of Cruelty to Children. Routledge & Kegan Paul, London

Department of Health 1991 Working together. HMSO, London

Kempe R, Kempe H 1978 Child abuse. Fontana, London

Leach P 1997 Your baby and child, 3rd edn. Penguin, London

Open University 1989 Unit P554: Child abuse and neglect. Course materials. Open University Press

Further reading

■ Bray M 1991 Poppies on the rubbish heap: sexual abuse: the child's voice. Canongate, Edinburgh

■ Butler-Sloss E 1987 Report of the inquiry into child abuse in Cleveland. HMSO, London

■ Campbell B 1988 Unofficial secrets, child sex abuse: the Cleveland case. Virago, London

■ Child Accident Prevention Trust 1994 Accident prevention in day care and play settings: a practical guide. Child Accident Prevention Trust, London

■ Children's Legal Centre 1988 Child abuse procedures: the children's viewpoint. Children's Legal Centre, London

■ Elliott M 1991 Feeling happy, feeling safe: a safety guide for young children. Hodder & Stoughton, London

■ Griffin S 1994 Keeping and writing records: a step-by-step guide for early years workers. VOLCUF Starting Points No 17, VOLCUF, London

■ Leach P 1992 Young children under stress. VOLCUF Starting Points No 13, VOLCUF, London

■ O'Hagan M, Smith M 1993 Special issues in child care. Baillière Tindall, London

■ O'Hagan M, Smith M 1999 Early years childcare and education: key issues. Baillière Tindall, London

■ VOLCUF 1990 Child abuse: a guide for under fives workers. VOLCUF, London

■ Wolfe L 1993 Safe and sound: a complete guide to first aid and emergency treatment for children and young adults. Hodder & Stoughton, London

Chapter 4

Diet and Nutrition

This chapter covers underpinning knowledge for parts of the following unit for the National Vocational Qualifications (NVQs) in Early Years Care and Education: C2. It is also linked to the following CACHE Awards Units: Diploma Unit 3; Certificate Unit 1.

INTRODUCTION

It is essential for children to have a well balanced diet if they are to thrive and develop physically and intellectually. The food that we eat supplies the essential nutrients needed for energy and growth. In recent years emphasis has been placed upon the healthy diet, with high profile media attention being given to healthy eating. Many more people are turning to vegetarianism for environmental or economic reasons and it is not uncommon to find children coming into nursery or school who are vegetarians for non-religious reasons. Parents are now more aware about the food that they give to their children and the harmful effects of so-called 'junk' foods. However, we live in a 'fast food' society where it is often cheaper and easier to buy a ready prepared meal than purchase the individual ingredients to make the same meal at home. In our society good food is expensive and a child's diet is likely to reflect the income of the family. Poor families may be forced to opt for the less nutritious but more filling foods such as bread, cakes and biscuits because these are cheaper. Purchasing the ingredients to make the food is just one aspect of producing the meal as it will still need to be cooked, and the prices of gas and electricity are high. Whilst it is cheaper to buy ready made frozen meals it is also cheaper to reheat these using a microwave oven. What would take 45 minutes to reheat in a conventional oven will only take 3 minutes on high power in a microwave oven. Microwave ovens are very useful when preparing a healthy but cheap diet, e.g. baked potatoes in their jackets are cooked very rapidly in a microwave oven.

Research carried out by Dobson et al (1994) interviewed families living on low incomes and the process by which these families decided what foods to eat. The following are some of the findings from this research.

■ Families changed their food-buying habits in order to economize. The cost of food took precedence over taste, cultural acceptability and healthy eating.

■ Mothers had to ration their supplies, decide where to shop, and not give in to temptation. Shopping became unenjoyable and they derived little pleasure from eating.

■ Families tended to shop little and often at local discount supermarkets.

■ Parents were concerned that their children should not be seen as different from their peer group and in order to maintain this gave them crisps or chocolate to take to school.

Whilst 'junk' foods such as crisps, chips, soft drinks, sweets and biscuits are harmful to children's teeth and may lead to overweight, there have been good cases made by nutritionists that pizzas, hamburgers, fish fingers etc. are not harmful to children.

Most child care establishments now take a great deal of care over the menus which they devise for the children in order to ensure that, whilst offering a well balanced diet, they also take into account children's preferences, the popularity of ethnic foods and the provision of vegetarian meals which appeal to children's tastes.

Britain is a pluralistic society and this is now reflected in the diet of many families. Dishes such as pizzas, curries, Chinese spare ribs, stir-fry vegetables, spaghetti, lasagne etc. are popular and feature very largely in the ready meals which are available in the frozen food sections of stores. Children enjoy these meals, which offer healthy alternatives to crisps, burgers, fish fingers and chips.

NUTRITIONAL INFORMATION

Calories

All foods contain calories, although different types of food will have different calorific values (see Table 4.1). A calorie represents the amount of energy that is produced when the body burns up the food. A calorie is a standard unit for measuring heat. It is the amount of heat energy required to raise the temperature of 1 g of water by 1°C. A kilocalorie is equal to the amount of heat energy required to raise the temperature of 1 kg of water by 1°C. Any surplus calorie intake that is not converted to energy remains in the body, leading to overweight.

Insufficient calorie intake will lead to the body not having enough calories to form the energy that is needed, and when this happens the body will draw upon its reserves to supply the energy, which results in weight loss. A child aged 2 years requires about 1000–2000 calories per day (Duff 1994).

Nutrient	Energy supplied per gram
Carbohydrate	4 kcal
Protein	4 kcal
Fat	9 kcal

Table 4.1 Energy value of food

Water

Water is essential to life in both the plant and animal world. Water is a component of every cell. In humans, water is needed to transport elements to cells, for the removal of body waste and to aid digestion. Some water is present in the food we eat but the greatest source of water for the body is drinking water, coffee, tea, milk, soft drinks etc. A lack of water leads to dehydration, a very serious condition for small babies and young children which, if untreated, can result in death.

Protein

Proteins provide the body with the essential amino acids, which are required for growth, repair of tissue and the production of antibodies, hormones and enzymes. Animal protein is the commonest source of protein in meat-eating societies. Vegetable proteins found in pulses/legumes such as lentils, peas, beans (e.g. soya, mung daal) and chick peas do not contain all the required amino acids; they are also less digestible and need to be consumed in much larger quantities in order to obtain the same amount of amino acids as would be supplied by animal protein. It is therefore important that careful attention is given to children on vegetarian diets to ensure that they receive an adequate intake of protein.

Other foods which are a source of protein are milk (casein), eggs, cheese and fish.

Lack of protein in the diet can lead to Marasmus, Kwashiorkor.

Carbohydrates

These are energy providing foods and they are stored in the liver in the form of glycogen. If there is too much carbohydrate in the diet to be stored as glycogen the remainder becomes body fat. Foods

SCENARIO 4.1

Mary is a childminder and has just agreed to care for Ranjit aged $2\frac{1}{2}$ years. Ranjit's family are members of the Hindu religion, although both his mother and father were born in the UK. What information will Mary need to obtain from Ranjit's parents about his diet and eating habits in order to ensure that he has an easy transition from home to childminder?

which are sources of carbohydrates are milk (lactose) and the 'starchy' foods such as cereals, pasta, bread, cakes etc. One of the greatest sources of carbohydrates is sugar and sweet foods. Too much sugar in the diet can lead to tooth decay and overweight.

Fats

These have a high calorific value in small quantities so are a good source of energy. Fats are essential as carriers of the fat-soluble vitamins (A, D, E, K); however, excess fat in the diet can lead to heart disease and obesity. Health educationalists make clear distinctions between the dangers of saturated fats, which are those found in meat and dairy products, and the healthier monounsaturated fats which are found in olive and rapeseed oil and polyunsaturated fats which are found in vegetable oils, fish oils, margarine etc. Duff (1994c) points out that the Department of Health recommends that fat should only be 30% of the total energy food intake and of this, 10% should be saturated fats, 12% should be monounsaturated fats and 6% should be polyunsaturated fats.

Fibre

Dietary fibre is highest in the following foods: bran, wholemeal bread, the fibrous parts of vegetables and fruit, root vegetables, peas, beans and cereals which have not been refined. Fibre is required in the diet in order to give bulk to food, as it is the part of food which is not digested by the body. Fibre stimulates the bowel action and prevents constipation, provided that additional fluid intake accompanies any additional fibre that may be added to the diet. However, it is pointed out by the DHSS (1988) that high fibre diets are not recommended for children under 5 years.

Vitamins

These are essential for growth and maintenance of the body. They cannot be manufactured by the body (except vitamin D) and so need to be obtained from the food that we eat. There are two types of vitamins:

- Fat soluble (A, D, E, K)
- Water soluble (B, C).

Vitamin A

Excess is stored in the liver.

- *Essential for:* good vision, healthy skin, formation of tooth enamel, resistance to infection
- *Sources:* liver, butter, whole milk, egg yolks, green vegetables, carrots, ripe tomatoes, fish liver oils, fortified margarine, apricots

■ *Symptoms of deficiency:* night glare and night blindness, rough scaly skin, poor tooth formation, eye inflammations.

Vitamin B complex

There are a number of vitamins in the vitamin B group:

■ Vitamin B_1 (thiamine)
■ Vitamin B_2 (riboflavin)
■ Vitamin B_3 (nicotinic acid)
■ Vitamin B_6 (pyridoxine)
■ Vitamin B_{12} (cyanocobalamin)
■ Folic acid.

Each of the above has a different chemical structure but acts in a similar way in the body. Vitamin B is used by the body to utilize proteins, carbohydrates and fats. Vitamin B is water soluble and is not stored in the body, any excess being excreted in the urine. Only the two most commonly known B vitamins (B_1 and B_2) will be looked at in any detail.

Vitamin B_1 (thiamine)

■ *Essential for:* functioning of nervous tissue, production of enzyme that uses carbohydrates
■ *Sources:* wholegrain cereals, nuts, peanut butter, eggs, wholemeal bread, milk and dairy foods, wheatgerm/brewer's yeast
■ *Symptoms of deficiency:* fatigue, constipation, depression, irritability and beriberi.

Vitamin B_2 (riboflavin)

■ *Essential for:* same as for B_1
■ *Sources:* milk, dairy foods, liver, meat, pulses/legumes, eggs, whole grain cereals, green leafy vegetables, wheatgerm/brewer's yeast
■ *Symptoms of deficiency:* burning/itching eyes, blurred/dimmed vision, eyes sensitive to the light, inflammation of the lips and tongue, greasy/scaly skin.

Vitamin C

It is water soluble and can be destroyed by heat.

■ *Essential for:* formation of teeth, bones and blood vessels, growth, healthy connective tissue
■ *Sources:* fresh fruit (especially citrus fruits and blackcurrants), fruit juices, tomatoes, vegetables (especially raw green) e.g. cabbage, broccoli, peppers, potatoes

■ *Symptoms of deficiency:* scurvy (sore mouth, stiff aching joints, lassitude), impaired wound healing, bleeding gums.

Vitamin D

It is fat soluble and is stored in the liver.

■ *Essential for:* absorption of calcium and phosphorus which are needed for the formation of bones and teeth
■ *Sources:* animal only – fatty fish such as halibut or cod, fish liver oils, egg yolk; it is added to margarine. Vitamin D can also be obtained from the action of sunlight on a substance in the skin called ergosterol
■ *Symptoms of deficiency:* rickets/osteomalacia, poor tooth development, bowed legs, soft bones.

Vitamin E

The functions of this vitamin are not fully understood. It is fat soluble.

■ *Sources:* vegetable oils, green leafy vegetables, egg yolk, milk fat, nuts, wheatgerm
■ *Symptoms of deficiency:* as the functions of vitamin E are unknown it is not possible to diagnose a deficiency.

Vitamin K

It is fat soluble and can only be absorbed if bile salts are present.

■ *Essential for:* the clotting process of the blood
■ *Sources:* green leafy vegetables, cauliflower, liver, soya bean oil
■ *Symptoms of deficiency:* haemorrhagic disease of the newborn, prolonged blood clotting time.

Minerals

These are elements, other than carbon, hydrogen and oxygen, which are essential for all bodily functions and growth and development. There are seven essential minerals: calcium, iodine, iron, phosphorus, potassium, sodium and zinc. The most likely of these to be lacking in the diet are calcium, iron, iodine and possibly zinc.

SCENARIO 4.2

David is a nursery officer in the toddler room of an inner city community nursery. David has recently noticed that Philip aged 2 years has been refusing to eat his lunch. What should David do to find out the cause of Philip's lack of appetite and how can he help Phillip regain an interest in food?

Calcium
- *Essential for:* healthy bones and teeth (in association with vitamin D and phosphorus), also the clotting process of blood
- *Sources:* milk, cheese, mustard, broccoli, cauliflower, cabbage, molasses, clams, oysters
- *Symptoms of deficiency:* rickets/osteomalacia, porous bones, bowed legs, stunted growth, tetany.

Iodine
- *Essential for:* production of thyroxine in the thyroid gland
- *Sources:* iodized salt, seaweeds, sea foods, vegetables grown in regions close to the sea
- *Symptoms of deficiency:* enlarged thyroid gland (goitre), low metabolic rate, stunted growth, retarded mental growth.

Iron

Absorption of iron is aided by vitamin C. Babies are born with a store of iron in their liver.

- *Essential for:* formation of haemoglobin in the blood
- *Sources:* red meat, liver, green vegetables, prunes, raisins, egg yolk, potatoes, wholegrain cereals, curry powder, sardines, haddock, cocoa
- *Symptoms of deficiency:* nutritional anaemia, pallor, weight loss, fatigue, weakness, retarded growth.

Phosphorus

Works in conjunction with Vitamin D and calcium.

- *Essential for:* maintenance of body fluids, cell structure, formation of bones and teeth
- *Sources:* milk, cheese, egg yolk, fish, nuts, pulses/legumes, wholegrain cereals
- *Symptoms of deficiency:* rickets/osteomalacia, porous bones, bowed legs, stunted growth.

Potassium

Works with sodium and can be lost during bouts of severe diarrhoea or if diuretics are used.

- *Essential for:* maintenance of body fluids
- *Sources:* wholegrain cereals, meat, potatoes, pulses/legumes, liver, fish, yeast extract, milk chocolate
- *Symptoms of deficiency:* apathy, muscular weakness, cardiac arrest, tachycardia (fast pulse rate).

Sodium

Babies cannot tolerate a high sodium intake due to the immaturity of their kidneys, therefore extra salt should never be added to their diet.

- *Essential for:* maintenance of cellular fluid, part of plasma, sweat and tears
- *Sources:* table salt, baking powder, milk, cheese, meat, egg white
- *Symptoms of deficiency:* dehydration, muscle cramps, weakness, headache, nausea
- *Symptoms of excess:* retention of water, changes in blood pressure, kidney damage.

Zinc

- *Essential for:* cell growth, healing of wounds; also controls activity of 100 enzymes and is involved in the functioning of insulin
- *Sources:* lean meat, wholewheat bread, wholegrain cereals, pulses/legumes, seafood
- *Symptoms of deficiency:* poor growth, delayed sexual maturation, impairment of taste, loss of appetite, hair loss, inflammation of skin, mouth and tongue; a deficiency may be caused by a malabsorption disease.

Healthy Eating and Food Groups

In order to have a healthy diet food from different groups needs to be chosen in particular proportions so that there is a correct distribution during a 24 hour period.

Potatoes and Cereals

These are foods which provide high levels of energy and include potatoes, pasta, rice, bread and cereals. They should be included in every meal; however, they need to be in direct proportion to the other food groups in the meal. Diets that are high in cereals and potatoes and low in other groups can lead to overweight when children do not get enough exercise.

Fruit and vegetables

These foods are high in vitamins and minerals and also offer fibre in the diet. They include carrots, tomatoes, oranges, grapefruits, celery etc. They are more nutritious if eaten raw but may be cooked (not over cooked as it destroys the vitamin content). A portion of fruit and vegetables should be included in every meal.

Milk and milk products

These are foods that have a high calcium content, which is essential for the growth of bones. They include, milk, yoghurt, cheese, fromage frais. Although these are also high fat content foods, children should not be given the low fat versions as they need the extra fat provided to give them energy. All children should have at least 250 mls of milk a day and a small portion of cheese (raw or cooked).

High protein foods	As their name suggests, these foods are a good source of protein which is essential for growth and repair of body tissue. Foods in this group are fish, poultry, eggs, lean meat, peas, beans (of numerous kinds), lentils, nuts and vegetarian products such as soya cake (tofu). Two helpings of this food group per day are sufficient for a well balanced diet.
Fats and oils	As these are found in all the other food groups there is no need for these to be added to the diet as a separate item.
	It is not necessary to add sugar or salt to a child's diet; in fact it can be very dangerous to add salt as young children's kidneys are unable to tolerate a high salt intake.
Additives	An additive is anything which is put into food that does not have a nutritional value, for example preservatives, flavourings, flavour enhancers, colourings, thickeners, stabilizers, emulsifiers, antioxidants and sweeteners. There are over 3000 additives available to British food manufacturers. The reason that manufacturers add these to food is to make the food more attractive to the purchaser. Polunin (1984) states that additives can be put into the following groups:

1. Built-in additives such as the addition of artificial sweeteners in low calorie drinks
2. Convenience additives which make life easier for the producer as they increase the shelf-life of the product. Examples of these are the preservatives added to meat pies, and anti-mould additives in bread
3. Cosmetic additives which help the product to be more attractive to the purchaser in appearance, taste, flavour, consistency etc. A large proportion of additives in this group are colourings, flavourings, flavour enhancers etc.

In the UK, additives to food are regulated by the Ministry of Agriculture, Fisheries and Food (MAFF) and have to comply with the Food and Drugs Act and other regulations. In line with the rest of the European Union (EU) all food packages must show the name and EU number of the additives. Thus if you are reading the ingredients on a packet you may also see 'tartrazine E102' (a food colouring), and 'sulphur dioxide E220' (a very common preservative). In recent years there have been a number of claims by researchers that there is an association between additives in food and hyperactivity in children. This idea was first put forward by Feingold in the USA, who suggested that children with over activity, short attention spans and impulsive behaviour might improve if they were given a diet which did not contain artificial colourings. Although scientists have yet to prove a causal relationship between food additives and hyperactivity, research carried out at Great Ormond Street Hospital does suggest that food additives such as tartrazine (E102), sulphur dioxide (E220), benzoic acid (E211, E212, E213) and monosodium glutamate (E621) could be associated with allergic conditions such as asthma, rashes, rhinitis and headaches.

Most parents and child care workers are aware of the possible dangers of additives and deliberately buy food and drinks for their children that do not contain numbers such as E102, E220, E211, E212, E213 and E621.

FOOD ALLERGIES

In recent years there has been a great deal of publicity about the dangers of food allergies to children. Peanuts and other nuts have proved to be particularly dangerous, leading to children suffering from anaphylactic shock, which if not treated quickly will result in death. As a consequence food manufacturers are now having to state very clearly on labels when a food product contains nuts. Less dangerous allergies to food or food additives can result in rashes, diarrhoea, vomiting etc.

CULTURAL/ DIETARY REQUIREMENTS

As previously mentioned in this book the UK is now a pluralistic society and as such a large number of early years settings will have children from a variety of cultural backgrounds. Whilst dietary requirements are mostly based upon religious requirements, much of what is eaten in a household, whether religious or non-religious, will relate to the cultural background of the household. Children will have a fondness for the food which they eat at home and it is therefore reassuring for them to find the same foods are on offer at the nursery or school. Most people are now familiar with dishes from many cultures; curries, pizza, pasta and noodles figure in many peoples' daily lives, as do tropical fruits and vegetables such as kiwis, dates, aubergines, courgettes etc. Parents/carers will be responsible for informing the establishment of their child's particular dietary likes and dislikes. Sometimes this does not happen and a child care worker may need dietary knowledge in order to ensure that a child is not inadvertently given food that it should not be eating. However, if a child care worker is ever in doubt about a child's diet it is best to offer a vegetarian meal. The following are some examples of the dietary requirements of different cultural/religious groups.

Jews

Jewish children are not allowed to eat any pork or pork products, or shellfish or fish that do not have fins and scales. There are also dietary laws relating to the mixing of milk and meat during a meal. The food that Jews eat at home will have a special label to show that its preparation has either been supervised by a Rabbi or the manufacturer has been inspected by a Rabbi and been found to be adhering to all the requirements as laid down by the religion (this food is called kosher). It is unlikely that a child from a strictly religious Jewish home background will be in a nursery or school as the community have their own early years provision including child minders. However, you may have a Jewish child from a liberal religious home background and it is best to treat this child as a vegetarian as this will ensure that there is no problem relating to meat or mixing milk and meat.

Hindus

Very strict Hindu households will be vegetarian, some eating eggs and dairy products. Less strict Hindus will not eat beef. In the Indian sub-continent it also usual for people not to eat pork as the pig is seen as a very unclean animal; however this is a cultural rather than a religious requirement.

Muslims

Muslims do not eat pork or any pork products. Other meat that is eaten must be killed in a certain way and this is called halal. Muslims do not eat shellfish or fish that do not have fins or scales.

Sikhs

Sikhs do not eat pork or beef, neither will they eat meat that is killed in the halal way. Some very orthodox Sikhs are vegetarian but most Sikhs will eat chicken and fish.

Rastafarians

Most Rastafarians are vegetarian and only eat foods which are considered to be ital or natural foods. Therefore they do not eat food which has been processed or pre-made.

Vegetarians

Vegetarianism has become very popular in the UK in recent years. This has been due in part to a number of food scares such as salmonella in chickens, 'Mad Cow Disease' (CJD), genetically modified foods etc. Added to this are the large numbers of people who are concerned over animal rights issues. Many aware parents have been particularly vigilant about the food their children are eating. Some vegetarians will eat eggs, fish and dairy products whereas vegans will not eat any food that is of animal origin. It is important to check with the parents and carers exactly which type of vegetarian group they wish their child to come under. There has been controversy relating to children under five having a totally vegan diet as they do need to eat an awful lot of pulses (beans such as soya, lentils, kidney beans etc.) in order to get the daily requirement of protein.

MEALTIMES

Mealtimes are part of the nursery and family routine and should happen at set times every day. There should be a pre-mealtime routine whereby the toys are packed away, children visit the toilet, wash their hands and then prior to eating may have a quiet activity such as a story. Once children are old enough they should participate in helping to lay the table ready for the meal. This activity is able to give them the mathematical experiences of learning about one-to-one correspondence, counting cutlery etc.

Mealtimes should be pleasant, relaxed social occasions for children with their family or at the nursery with their friends and carers. There should be plenty of time for children to feed themselves and enjoy their food in an unhurried atmosphere. Seating should be comfortable and of the right height to enable the child to reach the table. Eating utensils should be of a size and form which the child can manage. Children must always be encouraged to sit down and eat, a situation that some children may not be familiar with if they come from a home that relies on snack meals and 'TV dinners'. A good way to encourage children to develop social skills and table manners is for the child care worker to sit with the children and set an example of how they should behave at mealtimes. This also

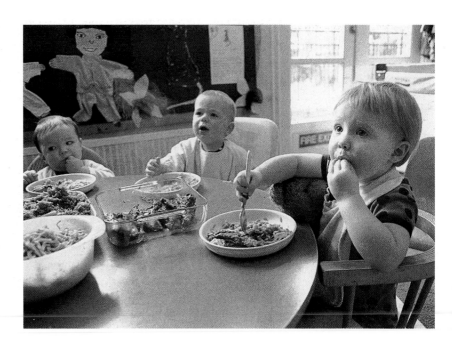

enables the child care worker to have the children who are difficult eaters sitting near her so she can offer help and encouragement. It is useful to remember that there are different cultural aspects to mealtimes, for example not all cultures use cutlery for eating, and using the fingers should not be frowned upon. In some cultures men and women eat separately, or children may sit together at a separate table from the adults. However, as children get used to the nursery they will want to do the same things as their friends and this will include copying the dominant eating habits.

Mealtimes are good opportunities for children to learn new skills and develop their language, through talking about the food that is being eaten, names of vegetables, meat, fish etc. Food also introduces children to different textures and colours. New words such as smooth, lumpy, chewy, hard, soft, cooked, raw, sweet, sour etc. all help to extend children's vocabulary and enable them to have a better understanding of their environment.

Meals should be served in an attractive manner and should contain a variety of tastes. If offering new foods to a child it is best to do this at the beginning of the meal when the child is hungry. Small portions of a new food can be introduced on a daily basis for a period of a week to enable the child to gradually get used to the taste. Small children like finger foods and this is a way of introducing raw vegetables, fruit, wholemeal bread etc. into their diet. Some children only like very small portions of food and this should be respected; the child care worker should only give them the quantity which they are happy with.

Children should be discouraged from eating snacks between meals as this takes away their appetite for the main meal. Many toddlers and pre-school children develop 'food fads', refusing to eat some foods or requesting the same food at every meal. There is no need to be alarmed at this as it is the child's way of gaining some independence and being able to choose what he will eat. Children should never be made to eat a food that they dislike or be force fed.

When devising menus for the nursery the children's cultural and religious backgrounds need to be taken into consideration. If you are working in a multi-cultural setting it is always wise to include a vegetarian dish on the menu. However, as previously mentioned, many families are vegetarian for reasons other than religion and these parents would also expect a vegetarian meal to be available for their children.

When children start at nursery it is useful to find out from parents what their dietary requirements are, including the foods that they like and dislike. It can also be useful to gain some knowledge from the parents as to what mealtimes are like in the home: are they used to sitting at a table, do they use a high chair etc. Some children may have food allergies, and child care workers need to be aware of these so they can ensure that the children are not offered the foods that cause the allergy.

SCENARIO 4.3

Pat is a playgroup leader. Every day the children arrive at playgroup with crisps, sweets and other snacks. Pat is worried that the children are eating too much 'junk' food during the playgroup session. What strategies can Pat use for dealing with this?

There may be children with special needs in the nursery and they may need special cutlery and equipment to help them eat independently. Equipment such as cups with specially shaped feeder spouts, cutlery with chubby shaped handles, or special chairs that enable them to reach the table may be required, depending upon the special needs of the child. These children must be given every opportunity and encouragement to learn to feed themselves, even if this means that for them mealtimes are a slow process.

FOOD HYGIENE

All people involved in the preparing of food or drinks for others who are not members of their family are required by the Food Safety Act 1990 to have a Food Handling Certificate. This is a very basic course which covers the main points attached to the hygiene of preparing and storing food. All childminders, playgroup workers and child care workers will need to gain this certificate. Environmental Health Officers from the local authority have the right to inspect all establishments where food and drinks are prepared and served.

Care should be taken in the handling of all food as bacteria can be found in cooked and uncooked foods. Most people in the UK have refrigerators for storing food; however, it is important to ensure that they are set at the correct setting so that food is stored at the right temperature. Modern fridges have an indicator inside which tells you if they are too warm. Cooked meats should be stored on the top shelves and raw meats on the bottom shelves to prevent contamination. Fresh food stored in a refrigerator should always be covered. Fridges should be defrosted regularly and thoroughly washed.

In Europe pre-packaged foods will have a number of dates printed on them, for example a 'sell by' date, a 'best before' date and a 'use by' date. When buying food always check that it has not passed its 'sell by' date. Do not use food that has passed the 'use by' date. Food that is marked with a 'best before' date can be used after the date is passed but will probably not taste as good, as the quality may have deteriorated. Some stores reduce foods on the day of the 'sell by' date; if these are purchased they should not be stored but used immediately.

Certain foods have gained a reputation for being carriers of salmonella or other types of food poisoning if they are not fully cooked, eggs and chicken being the main culprits. Raw eggs should not be given to babies, young children or other vulnerable people such as the sick or elderly. All chicken should be thoroughly cooked and particular care should be taken to ensure that the meat is cooked through to the centre. All frozen foods should be thoroughly defrosted before cooking. The use of microwave ovens has become commonplace; however, it is essential to ensure that all microwave meals are cooked all the way through. Microwave ovens come in different power strengths and it is important to ensure that the cooking time used is the right length for the power of the oven. Most microwave meals have full cooking instructions on the back of the packet. Microwaving makes food very, very hot and care must be taken to ensure that it is cooled before giving the meal to children.

Personal hygiene is important when handling food. Hands should be thoroughly washed before touching food. Any cuts or other open wounds should be covered with a waterproof dressing. The kitchen where food is prepared requires a high standard of hygiene. All surfaces should be washed down regularly using a disinfectant. Chopping boards should be colour coded, with separate boards for meat and vegetables. Wooden chopping boards must be thoroughly scrubbed with a brush and detergent after every use. All cutlery, crockery and cooking utensils should be washed after use in hot soapy water, rinsed and then dried thoroughly before storing. Rubbish bins should be emptied and cleaned regularly. It is important to keep the kitchen free from flies, which contaminate the food that they come to rest on. If food is prepared in advance and left on work surfaces then it should be covered to prevent contamination.

With the present day intensive farming methods many fruits and vegetables will have come into contact with fertilizers and other chemicals. It is therefore important to wash them before use. Some fruit, such as apples and lemons, are given a coating of wax in order for them to look more attractive; it is important that this is removed by thorough washing before they are given to children to eat.

ASSIGNMENTS

1. Plan a week's menus for your nursery bearing in mind that there are children who are vegetarians, Muslims and Afro-Caribbeans.

2. What is a balanced diet? Give a full explanation of what you understand by this term and what strategies you can use as a child care worker to ensure that the children in your care receive a balanced diet.

3. Scurvy was the curse of sailors in the 17th and 18th centuries. Why do you think this disease was so prevalent amongst this group of people? What components of the daily diet in present times go towards preventing scurvy?

4. By law all pre-packaged foods must have a breakdown of their components printed on the packet. What type of components are you likely to find that may be harmful to children if eaten regularly over a long period of time? State why you have chosen a particular component and the reasons for it being harmful.

5. Devise a project for a group of 4 year olds, which will make them more aware of the meaning of healthy eating.

6. Describe how a nursery cookery session could help children have a greater understanding of their diet.

PRACTICAL ACTIVITIES

1. Collect the menus for one week in your establishment and draw a graph showing the number of cultural meals that were offered and the number of vegetarian meals that were offered against the number of traditional UK meals that were offered. Discuss your findings with your superior.

2. Observe two children of a similar age group in your setting during meal times. Compare and contrast the observations and evaluate how their behaviour fits in with their developmental stage/s.

3. Organize an outing with two children from your establishment to the local greengrocer. List the new words which the children learned on the visit and describe how you will follow up this visit back in the establishment.

4. Draw up a policy for your setting about what happens when children bring sweets and crisps to the establishment and how this should be dealt with.

5. Observe a child who is a fussy eater. Draw up a plan as to how you intend to help the child over the next two weeks.

References

Department of Health and Social Security 1988
Present day practice in infant feeding. Report on
health and social subjects No 32. HMSO, London

Dobson B, Beardsworth A, Keil T, Walker R 1994
Eating on a low income. Social policy research No
66. Joseph Rowntree Foundation, York

Duff E 1994 On the sugar trail. Nursery World 29
September:26

Hilton T, Messenger M 1993 The Great Ormand Street
book of baby and child care. Bodlay Head,
Cambridge

Polunin M 1984 The right way to eat. Dent & Sons,
London

Further reading

- Burgess L 1995 Cookery activities. Bright
  ideas for early years series. Scholastic,
  London

- Duff E 1994 Vitamins. Nursery World
  6 October:26

- Duff E 1994 Fat in children's diets. Nursery
  World 13 October:19

- Food Safety Advisory Centre 1993 Food
  safety questions and answers. Food Safety,
  Advisory Council, London

- Greenslade J 1994 Go with the flow
  (importance of water in the diet). Nursery
  World 14 April:18

- HMSO 1998 Manual of nutrition. HMSO,
  London

There are numerous articles on food and
nutrition in child care magazines and general
magazines, including the Sunday colour
supplements.

Chapter 5

Working with Babies

This chapter covers underpinning knowledge for parts of the following units for the National Vocational Qualifications (NVQs) in Early Years Care and Education: C12, C13; there may also be some material appropriate for C14. This chapter is also linked to the following CACHE Awards Units: Diploma Unit 7; Certificate Unit Option A and some parts of Units 2 and 3.

INTRODUCTION

Many jobs in the child care and education field do not require workers to have knowledge and experience with the 0–1 year age group. However, many jobs do require knowledge and understanding of the 0–1 year age group, for example, child minding, nannies, mother's helps, those working in settings that offer full day care where there is a baby room etc. During recent years there has been an increase in provision in the education sector for the 3–5 year age group and parents have taken advantage of this by opting to send their child to a nursery school or class. In turn this has led to the age range in nurseries and family centres falling. Many day care facilities will take children from as young as 6 months and this means that there is a need to train carers to work with this younger age range of children.

In order for a baby to feel secure it needs to be cared for by the same person or a small team of people, for example parents/childminder, parents/nanny or parents/nursery worker. If the carers of the baby are constantly changing this will lead to the child feeling insecure. As John Bowlby (1953) pointed out in his studies on maternal deprivation, it is necessary for a baby to form attachments (bonding) with its carers and if this does not happen it may be detrimental to the child's development. The reason for a baby failing to bond may be the lack of opportunity for the child to do this due to the absence of stable caring figures, or to constantly changing carers. A baby can bond to a number of significant people in its immediate family group such as mother, father, siblings, grandparents, aunts, uncles etc. and in addition may also form attachments with the childminder, nanny or carer. As long as these people are constant figures in the baby's life they will be able to offer consistency and continuity of care. In the early days, babies are able to identify their carers by the way they hold them, the sound of their voice and the smell of the person.

There is a myth in society that caring for babies is just about feeding, changing nappies and putting the baby down to sleep. How wrong this analysis is. The first year of life is a period of rapid growth and development physically, socially, intellectually and emotionally. It therefore takes a special person to care for a baby, someone who is able to understand and respond to the baby's verbal and non-verbal messages, someone who is able to stimulate the child so that it is able to make its first movements towards sitting and walking, make the first coos and babbles towards language development etc. Therefore babies need carers whose role is to give them a safe secure environment, stimulation and loving care and attention.

For a family, the arrival of a new baby should be a joyous event for all members. The pregnancy is a time for preparation and coming to terms with the fact that there will be extra responsibilities for the adults. All members of the family should be involved in the preparations and siblings can be encouraged to feel the mother's stomach as the baby grows and help in choosing clothing, furniture and other items for the new baby. We live in a society where contraception and abortion are available and it should follow that all babies are wanted babies. Sadly, this is not always the case, for reasons, which may be very complex; not every baby will be wanted. Child care workers need to be aware of this as it may require them to work very hard to facilitate the bonding between a mother and her child.

Whilst most course syllabuses and the National Standards require a knowledge of babies, very few, if any, require the child care worker to have a knowledge of pregnancy and the birth of the baby. However, there is a certain illogic attached to only knowing about the baby once it is born, as what happens during pregnancy and the

SCENARIO 5.1

Sarah is on maternity leave with her first child, Siobhan. Sarah knows that in 6 weeks time she must return to work, therefore she is exploring all the available day care options in her locality. Sarah is worried about leaving Siobhan at such a young age for long periods of time, however, she has no alternative but to return to work. You are the Officer-in-Charge of the baby room in Sarah's local nursery. What would you tell Sarah about your provision that would reassure Sarah that she was doing the right thing by leaving Siobhan in your care?

birth process can have effects upon the way the mother feels about the baby and the future development of the baby. When child care workers discuss the baby with parents or carers they are likely to be expected to be familiar with the area relating to pregnancy and birth. This chapter covers these areas in some depth so that child care workers can feel confident that they have an understanding of pregnancy and birth.

PREGNANCY: SIGNS AND STAGES

Signs of pregnancy are missing a period or a change in the pattern of a woman's period. (Missing a period alone is not necessarily a sign of pregnancy; there may be other reasons for this happening.) 'Morning sickness', when the woman feels sick or is sick on getting out of bed in the mornings, is another sign. In some women this feeling of sickness and/or vomiting may occur at other times during the day. There may also be changes in the breasts, which may tingle or feel heavier with darkening around the nipple area. As the pregnancy progresses frequency in passing urine and tiredness are not uncommon symptoms. Confirmation of pregnancy is done through a simple test of the urine carried out by the GP. There are pregnancy testing kits which can be purchased from the chemist; however, these may vary in their accuracy. Once it has been confirmed that a woman is pregnant she will be advised to book into the ante-natal clinic in order to have her pregnancy monitored.

A normal pregnancy lasts for 40 weeks, and this is calculated from the first day of the woman's last menstrual period. Missing a menstrual period does not automatically mean that a woman is pregnant, therefore a doctor should be consulted for confirmation of pregnancy. There are home pregnancy testing kits which can be purchased at the pharmacists (chemists); however, these are not 100% accurate and there is always a risk that they will show the wrong result.

A woman's pregnancy is divided into three trimesters, each lasting for 3 months. In the first 8 weeks following conception the baby is referred to as an embryo. After that period it is called a fetus.

First Trimester (0–12 weeks)

First signs of pregnancy are the absence of menstrual periods. The breasts start to swell and become tender, the nipples start to enlarge. Nausea and vomiting are common and often occur in the morning (morning sickness); this may last for 6–8 weeks.

Second Trimester (13–28 weeks)

From about 16 weeks the enlarging uterus is easily felt and the woman begins to look noticeably pregnant. Nipples enlarge and darken. Appetite increases and weight can rise rapidly. By about the

22nd week the woman would have felt the baby moving around (quickening).

Third Trimester (29–40 weeks)

Stretch marks may begin to develop on the woman's abdomen. Colostrum can be expressed from the nipples. More rest may be needed at this stage. The baby's head engages (drops into the low pelvis) around the 36th week in preparation for the birth.

ANTE-NATAL CARE

The purpose of ante-natal care is to monitor the health of the mother and baby. If anything is found to be amiss with either the mother or the baby it can be dealt with quickly. Good ante-natal care provided free to all mothers is a major way of preventing and lowering the maternal and infant death rates.

On the first visit to the ante-natal clinic the woman will be able to discuss the available options for her ongoing care and the delivery of the baby. Depending upon the facilities available in the local health authority the woman may be able to choose between a home or hospital delivery, and whether her ante-natal care will be a shared responsibility between her GP, Community Midwife and hospital or will be totally the responsibility of the hospital. Nearer the time of her delivery the staff at the antenatal clinic will discuss with the woman the birth positions which may be available, for example crouching, birthing chairs, birthing pools, stirrup position etc. and the advantages and disadvantages of each. It will then be left for the woman to make up her mind and to inform the midwife of her preferences once she has gone into labour. Mothers are encouraged to actively involve their partners in the pregnancy and birth. If a woman is going through the pregnancy alone she will be encouraged to involve a close family member of friend who can act as a support for her during the ante-natal period and the birth.

Ante-natal clinics are also able to offer parentcraft classes and general advice to the mother and her partner about what is happening throughout the different stages of the pregnancy and what can be expected at the onset of labour. The first 12 weeks of pregnancy are, in many ways, the most critical as it is during this time that the baby's essential organs are being formed. Once a woman thinks that she is pregnant (although not necessarily confirmed by a doctor), it is important that she carefully considers changing any parts of her lifestyle which could be harmful to the baby. The following are examples of the things which an expectant mother may have to consider changing during pregnancy.

Smoking
It is now a well established scientific fact that smoking retards the growth of the fetus by cutting down the oxygen supply to the baby. Mothers who smoke when they are pregnant are more likely to have a low birthweight baby or a baby described as small for dates. These babies are very vulnerable and may need special care after birth. Women who smoke should do everything possible to give up smoking during the pregnancy. This will take a lot of willpower and the woman will need support from her family and friends. Many GP group practices have special clinics to help people give up smoking and she may find it easiest to attend one of these.

Alcohol
Excessive regular intake of alcoholic drinks by a woman who is pregnant can lead to a low birthweight baby. Alcohol in the bloodstream of the mother is able to cross the placenta and have an effect upon the development of the baby. Women who are alcoholics and who continue to drink during their pregnancy are at risk of having a baby which has fetal alcohol syndrome; this not only gives the child distinctive features but also leads to mental retardation.

Diet
Pregnant women need a well balanced diet. The old wives' saying of 'eating for two' is not helpful, as it is the quality of the food and type of food consumed which is important, not the quantity. During the pregnancy the woman should gain about 12.7 kg and 70% of this weight increase should occur during the last 20 weeks of the pregnancy. There should be a daily intake of each of the following: protein, fruit, vegetables, fats, dairy products, cereals and whole grains. There should also be an adequate fluid intake as this prevents constipation. If the woman has a well balanced diet she should not need any vitamin or mineral supplements except those advised by a doctor or midwife. Vegetarians who do not eat fish, eggs or cheese (vegans) need to take special care with their diet to ensure that their protein intake is of a higher level than they would normally need.

There are some foods which are best avoided during pregnancy as they may cause listeria or salmonella poisoning and this could be harmful to the baby. Pregnant women should avoid raw or lightly cooked eggs, undercooked chicken, rare or lightly cooked meat, soft cheeses (such as Brie, Camembert) or mould ripened cheeses (such as Stilton, Roquefort, Blue Brie).

Exercise
A normal amount of exercise is good for the health of the woman and the baby. However, it is not the time to take up jogging or

cycling! Swimming, walking or simple exercises done on a regular basis will help the woman to keep fit. Exercise also helps to prevent constipation. The ante-natal clinic will offer exercise classes but these are specifically related to the labour and post-labour period.

Dental Care

Dental treatment is free during pregnancy and up until the baby is 1 year old. The mother's dental health depends a great deal upon her diet, and foods rich in protein, calcium, phosphorus and vitamins A, C and D are important (the future teeth of the baby are laid down during the early months of pregnancy and therefore the mother's diet during this time will also affect the quality of the child's teeth). Teeth that are decaying can cause infections and these in turn might be harmful to the baby; it is therefore important that pregnant women take advantage of the free dental treatment which is offered to them.

Drugs

It is important that once a woman thinks that she may be pregnant she should stop taking any drugs, even those that have been prescribed for her. Women on a permanent drug regime, such as diabetics, asthmatics or epileptics, should consult their GP immediately. Doctors have a great deal of experience in monitoring women who are on permanent drug regimes. Drugs, like alcohol, are able to cross the placenta and could have serious harmful effects upon the baby.

Drug addicts who become pregnant must also contact their doctors who will be able to offer them advice and counselling to help them give up the drugs and may also be able to offer less potent substitutes for the hard drugs that the woman may be addicted to. It is not uncommon for babies who are born to drug addicts to suffer withdrawal symptoms following the birth.

X-rays

X-rays can be harmful to the developing fetus. In the majority of hospitals the radiographer, before taking an X-ray, will always check with female patients as to whether they think they could be pregnant. If a woman suspects that she might be pregnant and is sent for an X-ray she should always tell the radiographer.

Rubella (German Measles)

For a woman to contract rubella in the first trimester (3 months) of pregnancy can cause damage to the development of the fetus. Such damage may result in the baby being born deaf, blind or mentally or physically handicapped. Since 1970 there has been a vaccination programme in secondary schools in the UK whereby teenage girls are given rubella vaccine. This has led to a dramatic fall in the numbers of children being born with rubella-associated handicaps. However, it should be noted that any woman who did not have her secondary school education in the UK may not have had the benefit of this vaccine and should therefore be warned of the dangers of contracting rubella during pregnancy. For this reason, parents of children who contract rubella should make sure that all the adult females that the child has had contact with are made aware that the child has rubella.

ANTE-NATAL SCREENING

The Health of the Mother

On the first visit to the ante-natal clinic there will be a number of screening tests that will be carried out on the mother. At this stage of the pregnancy these will be done in order to ascertain the state of health of the mother.

Blood screening

On the first ante-natal visit a sample of the mother's blood will be taken. This will be screened for the following:

- Blood group
- Rhesus factor
- Syphilis
- Viral hepatitis
- Rubella immunity
- Sickle cell disease
- Thalassaemia
- Haemoglobin level
- AIDS/HIV (for those women who think they may have been at risk).

On the initial visit and subsequent visits the mother will also undergo urine screening.

Urine screening

A urine sample will be taken from the mother every time that she visits the ante-natal clinic. This sample will be tested for:

- Sugar
- Protein
- Ketones.

Blood pressure and weight will also be taken at each visit. If the woman registers a low haemoglobin count in the first blood test, further tests may be taken at subsequent ante-natal visits throughout the pregnancy.

Ultrasound Screening

Most pregnant women will be automatically given an ultrasound scan at around 16–18 weeks of the pregnancy. This test is done by transmitting high frequency sounds, which cannot be heard, to the womb (it is the same method that is used to detect submarines). As the sounds bounce back they can be captured on a screen to form a picture of the baby in the womb. This test is quite harmless to the mother and baby and does not cause discomfort or distress. Ultrasound scanning can confirm the number of weeks of the pregnancy, whether there is more than one baby, that the baby is lying in the womb and not outside it, i.e. in a fallopian tube, that the baby is developing normally and the position that the baby is lying in. The ultrasound scan can also determine the sex of the baby and this information can be given to the parents/family if they want to know. The sex of the baby can be important when there are inherited sex-linked conditions such as haemophilia or Duchenne's muscular dystrophy. Many hospitals are able to provide a photograph of the ultrasound scan picture so the family has a first picture of the baby.

Other Screening Tests

There are other screening tests which a pregnant woman may undergo at later dates during the pregnancy; these tests may be offered to all women or just to those who may be at risk. A woman has a choice as to whether she wishes to have these tests carried out. If the tests prove to be positive the woman then has the choice of continuing with the pregnancy or having it terminated (an abortion). If a woman has particular convictions about not wishing to have an abortion (these convictions may or may not be linked with religious beliefs) then she may not wish to have these tests carried out.

Spina bifida

This test may be offered as routine or to a woman who is in a high risk category, i.e. there is a history of spina bifida in the family or she already has a child with spina bifida. This test is carried out in the 16th week of the pregnancy. A blood sample is taken and tested for the level of alpha-fetoprotein (AFP) which may indicate that the child possibly has spina bifida. Low levels of AFP can also indicate that the child may have Down's syndrome.

Down's syndrome

The AFP test may be offered to women who are in a high risk category, i.e. over the age of 35 years, who already have a Down's syndrome child or where there is a history of Down's syndrome in the family. As already stated, low levels of AFP may indicate that the baby has Down's syndrome.

Amniocentesis This test is carried out between the 14th and 16th weeks of the pregnancy. Using the ultrasound picture to guide the direction, a needle is used to draw off a sample of the amniotic fluid (this is the fluid that surrounds the baby in the womb). The amniotic fluid will contain cells from the baby and these can be tested for Down's Syndrome and some other genetic disorders. There is a 0.05% risk of a spontaneous miscarriage following an amniocentesis test.

Chorion biopsy This test is carried out between the 7th and 11th weeks of the pregnancy. A sample of cells is taken from the chorionic villi which are found in the embryonic membrane (chorion). The sample of cells is then tested in order to detect genetic diseases such as cystic fibrosis, Duchenne's muscular dystrophy, haemophilia, thalassaemia etc. The test is offered to women from families where there is a history of these diseases.

SCENARIO 5.2

Sharon is your neighbours' 17-year-old daughter. Sharon is 3 months pregnant. On talking with Sharon you discover that she has not attended any of her ante-natal clinic appointments. How would you explain to Sharon about the importance of ante-natal care and how would you best convince her that she should attend these clinics?

Multiple births With ultrasound scanning it is now possible to detect at an early stage of the pregnancy the number of children that a woman is carrying. Fraternal twins are those formed when two eggs are fertilized at the same time, whereas identical twins are when one egg splits into two. Fraternal twins are more common than identical twins. With the latest treatments for infertility becoming more easily available there has been a proportional increase in the numbers of multiple births, particularly triplets and quads.

THE BIRTH By the time a woman goes into labour (the term used to describe the birth process, probably called this as giving birth is hard work!) she will know whether she is having the baby at home or in hospital. She would also have been instructed at the ante-natal clinic or by her midwife as to the first signs of the onset of labour such as contractions, or the breaking of the waters (amniotic fluid) and what to do when these occur. There are three stages to labour.

Stage 1

This is the stage of dilation of the cervix. It starts with regular uterine contractions which push the baby and the sac of amniotic fluid downwards and the uterus upwards. The cervix, uterus and vagina all dilate in order to provide one continuous birth canal. During this stage the amniotic sac may burst or this may not happen until later in the proceedings.

Stage 2

This stage extends until the baby is delivered. During this stage the baby is pushed through the birth canal. Every contraction brings the baby further forward. Once the baby's head is through the rest of the baby can be eased out.

Stage 3

This is the stage following the birth of the baby and during which the placenta is expelled and the uterus contracts. Following the expulsion of the placenta the uterus continues to contract and diminishes in size in order to control the bleeding. On average the whole birth process will take up to 14 hours for a first baby and 8 hours for each subsequent birth.

IMMEDIATELY FOLLOWING THE BIRTH (THE NEWBORN BABY)

The midwife will take care of the baby, cutting the umbilical cord at the beginning of the third stage of labour. The baby may have taken its first breath when the head emerges, but in some cases the midwife may have to extract mucus in the baby's mouth and throat in order to help it take this breath. The baby will be examined and given a rating known as the Apgar score (Table 5.1). This test is named after its inventor Virginia Apgar and records the heart rate,

Table 5.1 *The Apgar score*

Signs	Score		
	0	1	2
Heart rate[a]	Absent	Slow (below 100)	Fast (above 100)
Respiratory effect[a]	Absent	Slow Irregular	Good Crying
Muscle tone	Limp	Some limb movements	Active
Reflex irritability (stimulation of foot or nostril)	No response	Grimace	Cry, cough
Colour	Cyanosed (Blue) or very pale[b]	Good colour Limbs blue	Very good colour

[a] The first two, heart rate and respiratory effect, are the most important.
[b] In babies with black/dark skin tones it may be more difficult to see cyanosis (blueness) and lips and nailbeds are carefully examined. Midwives working in multi-cultural areas are very familiar with the differences in skin tones.

The three stages of labour. 1. Onset of contractions to full cervical dilatation (10 cm). 2. Full dilatation to delivery of infant. 3. Delivery of placenta or 'afterbirth'.

Stage 1

Stage 2

Stage 3

muscle tone, breathing and colour immediately following the birth. Babies with a low Apgar score (0–8) will be carefully monitored in the first few days following the birth. Babies without difficulties usually have an Apgar score of 8–10.

All newborn babies look different and they may or may not have some of the features mentioned below.

The skin of a newborn baby is covered with a greasy film called vernix. It used to be traditional in the UK to bath the baby immediately following birth in order to wash off the vernix. However, research has shown that the vernix is best left on the baby where it is absorbed through the skin and offers the baby protection against skin infections.

The baby's face may be wrinkled and red or puffy or in some cases bruised. All these marks will disappear within the first few days following the birth.

Some babies will have a good head of dark hair which grows downwards onto the forehead. In most babies the first hair, whatever the texture and colour, will fall out and the subsequent growth of hair may bear no resemblance to the birth hair. In some religions and cultures the hair that a baby is born with is thought to be unlucky or to sap the child's future strength. In these situations the family will shave off the birth hair; this does no harm to the baby.

The body of some babies may be covered in downy hairs which are shed after the baby is about a week old.

Once the midwife has checked the baby it will be wrapped up and given to the mother to hold. At this point some midwives will encourage the mother to put the baby to the breast.

EXAMINATION OF THE NEWBORN

In the first 24 hours following the birth a doctor will usually give the baby a thorough examination.

Basic Measurements

The length of the baby and the circumference of the baby's head is measured, and the baby is then weighed. The average weight of a newborn baby is 2.5–4.4 kg ($5\frac{1}{2}$ –$9\frac{1}{2}$ lb), the average length is 45–55 cm (18–22 inches) and the head circumference should be about 35 cm (14 inches). A baby may lose weight following the birth but the original birthweight should be regained by the tenth day.

Head and Neck

The doctor will check the fontanelle (soft spot) on the top of the head and check for any swelling (caput) on parts of the scalp caused by pressure during the birth.

The Face

The baby's face is examined in order to check for abnormalities such as a harelip or cleft palate, which would result in difficulties in feeding. The doctor will also check the fold of skin which holds the tongue to the floor of the mouth to ensure that it is not too short. Vision and hearing are checked by watching the child's response to light and sound.

The Heart

The heart is checked using a stethoscope. The doctor listens for abnormal heart sounds such as 'murmurs', and checks the baby's lips and nails for signs of cyanosis (blue colour), both of which could indicate that the child has a congenital heart condition.

The Genitals

The doctor inspects the genitals in order to confirm that the sex of the child has been correctly stated. Male children will also be tested to ascertain whether the testicles have descended into the scrotum.

The Umbilical Cord

The cord is checked to ensure that it is drying out normally and not becoming infected. It is not uncommon to find that some babies have a hernia around the cord area; this needs no treatment and usually disappears around the age of 5 years.

Congenital Dislocation of the Hip

The doctor is able to put both the hip joints through a range of movements to determine whether the baby has dislocated a hip during the birth process. This test does not hurt the baby. If a dislocated hip is diagnosed the baby will be referred to an orthopaedic specialist for treatment.

Hands and Feet

The hands and feet are examined for extra digits, webbing between the digits and any other deformities such as talipes (clubfoot).

Reflexes

A baby is born with a number of reflexes which will be tested by the doctor at the post-birth examination. These reflexes are simple responses to stimuli as follows:

- *Oral:* sucking
- *Rooting:* when the baby's cheek is touched at one side of the mouth it will turn its head to the touch
- *Eyes:* blink in response to light
- *Grasp:* will grasp a finger that is placed in the palm of its hand
- *Moro:* if the baby is startled it flings out its arms and opens its hands
- *Walking:* will attempt to walk when its feet come into contact with a horizontal surface.

Blood Tests

A routine blood test is taken from babies when they are 7 days old and this is used to screen for phenylketonuria (PKU) and is called the Guthrie test. A second test is carried out to determine the functioning of the baby's thyroid gland.

The reflex grasp and movements from lying to sitting of a newborn baby.

Pre-term Babies

Pre-term or premature babies are those that are born before week 37 of the pregnancy. These babies will have a low birthweight, often less than 2.3 kg; be small in size with a large head and hands; the skin will be thin, shiny, smooth and will be covered in downy hair (lanugo); features may be wizened and wrinkled; veins may be visible under the skin; the abdomen will protrude; they will have a poor sucking and swallowing ability and may have a feeble whining cry.

Pre-term babies are at risk from respiratory distress, jaundice, poor temperature control, anaemia, low blood sugar and infection. These babies are very vulnerable and will be cared for in the Special Care Baby Unit (SCBU) usually in an incubator. An incubator provides warmth and allows easy observation of the baby; it has artificial ventilation to assist breathing. These babies will probably need to be fed artificially through a stomach tube. They will be kept in the incubator until they reach a weight of 2.5 kg and must be able to feed normally. 90% of premature babies survive and are able to catch up with full term babies over a period of time.

Small-for-dates Babies

These are babies who have gone through the full period (40 weeks) of pregnancy but when born have a low birthweight, under 2.3 kg (5 lb). These babies may have breathing and feeding problems and some may need to be monitored in the Special Care Baby Unit for a period of time. These babies are often born to mothers who are heavy smokers, heavy drinkers or have had poor nutrition during pregnancy.

Abilities of the Newborn

Vision

Newborn babies are able to focus on an object that is at a distance of 8–9 inches from their eyes. This distance is the amount of space between a baby feeding on the breast and the face of the mother. Professor Karmiloff-Smith of the Medical Research Council Cognitive

Development Unit in London (see Reid 1995) has found that at 4 days old an infant can recognize its mother by the shape of her face and her hair. It would appear that babies have a primitive orientation, which allows them to distinguish between many different types of face. Infants gradually specialize in faces so that at the age of 2 months they prefer the whole face with all its features and at 5 months they like a moving face.

Hearing

Normally hearing babies will hear loud noises, which will lead them to respond by making the Moro reflex.

Smell

A baby has a sense of smell and can recognize the smell of its mother's milk.

Touch

Many of the reflex responses of the baby are in response to touch.

Language

Recent research by Professor Annette Karmiloff-Smith (see Reid 1995) has found that newborn babies can distinguish the sound of their parents'/carer's languages from other languages which they may hear. Professor Karmiloff-Smith maintains that newborn babies are capable of distinguishing between each of the 150 speech sounds that make up all human languages, although by the age of 10 months they have lost this sensitivity.

Birthmarks

Newborn babies often have marks on their skin, the majority of which will disappear during the first few months of life.

Stork's beak marks

This term is used to describe the small pink marks which a baby may have above the bridge of the nose, on the eyelids or the nape of the neck. These usually fade over time.

Strawberry marks

These are tiny red dots, which are not always obvious at first. They grow during the early months of life to become red raised lumps. They usually begin to shrink in the second year of life and may have totally disappeared by the time the child reaches school age.

Mongolian blue spot

This is the name given to a mark which is commonly found in Asian or black children but may also occur in children from other ethnic origins such as Italian, Greek, Oriental and Eskimo (Inuit). It is a blue discolouration of the skin usually found on the lower back. This will fade over time. It is important that this is recognized as a birthmark and is not confused with a sign of physical abuse.

Moles (pigmented naevus)

These may be brown or blackish, flat or raised and may or may not have hairs sprouting from them. They usually appear in places where they are hidden by clothing; however, if a child has a disfiguring naevus it can be removed by plastic surgery.

Port wine stain

Of all the birthmarks found on new babies this is one of the most serious, as it does not fade with time; however, it is comparatively rare. It appears as a dark red patch with sharply defined edges. It is a permanent mark and depending on where it appears may need to be dealt with in later life by the application of masking creams.

Spots and rashes

It is not uncommon for newborn babies to get spots and rashes, which are usually harmless and disappear after a short time. The most common two rashes are:

- *Neonatal urticaria:* These are large red spots, which may appear during the first week of life. They disappear after a few hours and others may appear in different places. They need no treatment and will eventually disappear altogether.
- *Milia:* These are small white spots usually appearing on the nose. They are caused through blocked sebaceous glands. They need no treatment and will disappear of their own accord.

SCENARIO 5.3

You are the Officer-in-Charge in the baby room of the local family centre. Shamila is an 8-month-old Asian girl in your care. Carol, the student child care worker, tells you that whilst she was changing Shamila she saw evidence of bruising on her back. What is the most likely explanation for what Carol has seen? How do you explain the situation to Carol?

FEEDING THE NEW BABY

Most mothers have a choice of breast feeding or bottle feeding their baby. However, some mothers may have physical problems which may prevent them breast feeding, e.g. needing to take drugs which will pass to the baby via the breast milk; or the baby may have physical problems which make breast feeding difficult, e.g. a cleft palate. In order for a woman to make an informed choice between breast feeding and bottle feeding the reasons for both need to be explained to her.

Reasons for breast feeding:

- Breast milk is a natural food, easily digestible for the baby and requires no vitamin supplements.
- Breast milk is always at the right temperature, requires no preparation, is always available to the baby and is cheap to provide.
- Breast milk contains antibodies which protect the baby against disease and infection.
- Breast milk is less likely to cause the baby to have allergic reactions.
- Breastfed babies are not usually overweight.
- Breast feeding helps the development of the baby's gums, teeth and jaws as the baby has to suck more vigorously in order to obtain the milk.
- Breast milk can be expressed so that babies can be given the milk in a bottle in order for the mother to have shared care of the baby. This may be particularly useful when there are twins or other multiple births.

Reasons for bottle feeding:

- Bottle feeding may make the mother feel more confident, particularly if she has had difficulties trying to breast feed.
- If the woman wishes to return to work soon after the birth it may be easier to bottlefeed the baby from the beginning.
- If it is a multiple birth situation, bottle feeding will enable others to be involved at feeding times which may make the process less stressful for the mother.
- Feeding can be shared between the mother and her partner.

Breast feeding is the recommended method of feeding a baby and most mothers are able to successfully establish breast feeding with their baby. However, there may be very valid reasons for a woman choosing to bottle feed her baby, and the wishes of the mother should be respected.

During the first weeks of life the baby and mother together will be establishing a feeding routine. In the first instance the baby may be fed on demand and gradually this will settle down into regular periods between feeds, usually a pattern that gives the baby four to six feeds a day.

Breast Feeding

Techniques to establish breast feeding are suggested by the midwife. This is very important for first time mothers as they may lack confidence in breast feeding their baby. It is important that the mother sits/lies in a position which is comfortable for herself and the baby. The baby should be held in a comfortable way ensuring that the back of the child's neck is supported. In order for the baby to express milk from the breast it needs to be 'fixed on' to the nipple and its surrounding area. The baby holds on by suction but feeds by moving its lower jaw up and down, squeezing the milk reservoirs which lie behind the nipple. The production of breast milk is on supply and demand regardless of the size of the breasts, therefore the more often the baby is put to the breast the more milk the breasts will produce. The baby should empty both breasts at each feed. If a baby is breast feeding satisfactorily it will fall asleep between feeds, gain approximately 140–225 g per week and pass soft yellow stools after the end of the first week (before this period the baby will pass what is called meconium, which is dark and sticky). Some babies take longer than others to learn to feed and the mother needs to be patient and gain advice and help from the midwife and health visitor. The La Leche League is a charitable organization, which provides information, encouragement and support to women who are breast feeding. The La Leche League runs a 24 hour helpline and has local meetings (address in Appendix).

It is important that before breast feeding a mother washes her hands. The breasts should be washed daily and if the nipples are sore a barrier cream should be applied. When the woman is breast feeding she will need a well balanced diet with plenty of liquids. She will also need to remember that whatever she takes into her body may come out in the breast milk so that strong-flavoured food such as garlic, pickled onions etc. may flavour the breast milk. Drugs and alcohol may also pass into the breast milk and the breast

A baby breast feeding. Note that the nipple is well back in the baby's mouth.

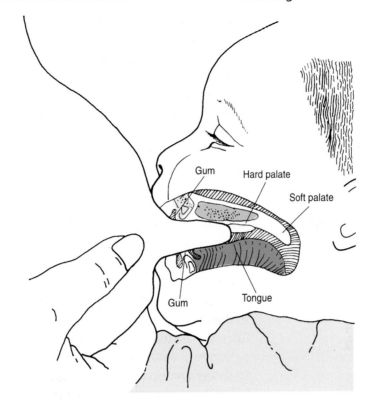

Gum

Hard palate

Soft palate

Gum

Tongue

feeding mother should take great care over things such as laxatives, aspirin, caffeine and nicotine.

Bottle Feeding

Babies under 6 months of age are unable to digest cow's milk. Unless the mother is expressing her own breast milk and bottle feeding her baby with this, she will need to decide which brand of dried milk formula she will use for her baby. This decision is best made in consultation with the midwife or health visitor. Most baby milk formulas are supplemented with vitamins A, B_{12}, C and D.

It is important that all the equipment used to make up bottle feeds and the bottles and teats are sterilized before use. There are a number of sterilizing agents available on the market and the instructions for using these should be followed carefully. A plastic sterilizing unit can be purchased and this will hold a number of bottles and teats. Metal implements cannot be sterilized using proprietary sterilizing agents so it is better to use plastic spoons, knives, or glass/Pyrex measuring jugs. In the absence of chemical sterilizing agents the equipment should be boiled in a saucepan of water, ensuring that all the equipment is fully submerged in the water and the water is kept at boiling temperature for at least 10 minutes. If this method of sterilization is used the equipment will need to be drained and allowed to cool naturally before using.

When preparing a feed using milk formula it is important to follow all the instructions which are printed on the packet. The scoop provided in the packet of milk must be used and a 'level scoop' is a scoop which has been levelled by passing a knife or other flat utensil across the top of the scoop. The scoop should be lightly filled (not packed full as this will make the feed too concentrated) and half scoop measures should not be used as they cannot be measured accurately. Sugar must not be added to the feed.

Preparing the feed

Nurseries will have a milk kitchen, which is an area separate from the main kitchen and used only for preparing bottle feeds. In the home, the person preparing the feed should use an area in the kitchen that is easy to keep scrupulously clean. When preparing a bottle feed, strict attention should be paid to cleanliness of the area where the feed is being made and to the good hygiene practices of the person preparing the feed.

Before making the feed all the necessary equipment should be gathered together. You will need the milk formula, boiled water and the following previously sterilized utensils: a plastic straight edged knife, glass/Pyrex jug, feeding bottle and teat. Always wash your hands before preparing the feed. Following the manufacturer's instructions on the milk formula packet, pour the required amount of boiled water into the jug, add the required amount of milk formula, stirring to ensure that there are no lumps, pour this into the feeding bottle, place the teat on the bottle and cover this with the teat protector. A variety of milk formulas can be made straight into the bottle/s without the need of a jug. The formula is measured and put into the bottle, the water is added using the measurements on the side of the bottle, the top is put onto the bottle and the bottle shaken vigorously in order to mix the contents. The feed that is made straight into a bottle will need to be cooled before it can be given to the baby. All the bottles needed to feed a baby for a 24 hour period can be made at the same time, storing them in the refrigerator and reheating using a microwave or a jug of hot water. It is only possible to use this method if the carer has enough bottles; feeds cannot be made in advance and kept in other containers until needed as this will lead to contamination of the feed. Place the bottle on a tray with two jugs of water, one hot and one cold. Take the tray to the room where you will be feeding the baby and place it in a safe position but within easy reach of the person who is feeding the baby. Always wash your hands before you feed a baby.

When feeding a baby it is best to sit it on your lap in a similar position to the one they would be in if they were being breast fed. *Babies must not be fed lying in cots or propped up in chairs.* Holding the baby close during feeding is part of the bonding process between the carer and child. The temperature of the milk must always be tested before giving the feed to the baby. This is done by putting a few drops of milk on the back of the adult's hand; it should not be too hot or too cold. If the feed is too hot the bottle should be placed in the jug of cold water until it cools to the right temperature. If the feed is too cold the bottle should be placed in the jug of hot water until it reaches the right temperature. If the feed is heated using a microwave it will still need to be cooled and the temperature tested before it is given to the baby. The size of the hole in the teat should enable the baby to get a free flow of milk when it sucks hard. If the hole is too large the baby will not have to suck so hard and will miss out on strengthening its jaw muscles. When feeding the baby the bottle should be held at an angle that ensures that there is no gap between the teat and the liquid. This prevents the baby sucking in air which can result in the baby getting 'wind'. All babies take in some air during the sucking process and it is a good idea to stop the feed half way through and 'wind' the baby. This is done by holding the baby in an upright position, usually supported on the shoulder of the person feeding the baby, and gently rubbing the baby's back until it burps (expels the air). This also needs to be done at the end of the feed. Air trapped in the baby's stomach can be painful. After feeding the baby should have a nappy change and be put into its cot to sleep.

Following the feed all the bottle feeding equipment needs to be thoroughly washed and placed into the sterilizing unit, making sure that the sterilizing fluid gets right inside the bottles and there are no air bubbles. Bottles need to be washed using a bottle brush and should be washed in cold water first to remove milk residues and film. The same care applies to teats. The sterilizing solution needs to be changed every 24 hours. Bottle-feeding utensils are a potential source of infection and must therefore be carefully washed and sterilized before using to prepare a feed. For babies, infections such as gastroenteritis are very serious and if not treated by a doctor immediately can lead to complications and even death.

Weaning

Weaning is the term used to describe the baby's transition from breast or bottle feeding to solid foods. (In some books it may also be used to describe the baby's transition from breast feeding to bottle feeding.) At about 4–6 months of age most babies will require more food intake than they can obtain from a milk-only diet. Bottle fed babies seem to give signs that they are dissatisfied with their feeds earlier than breast fed babies; this may be due to the fact that the harder a breast fed baby sucks the more milk there is available to it. Research by Dr Gill Harris from Birmingham University (see Reid 1995) has found that babies are most receptive to a wide range of foods between 3 and 6 months. In some cultures, babies are weaned at a much later date; this may be due to tradition, unavailability of suitable weaning foods, or economics, as breast milk is free. Research appears to show that the later a baby is weaned the less chance there is of the child having allergic reactions to certain foods. The common foods that may produce allergic reactions are cow's milk, eggs (particularly egg white), wheat, cheese, shellfish and pork.

Babies should never be weaned by adding cereals to their bottle feed. The foods that are used to wean a baby will vary depending upon the culture and diet within the family. For example, the Chinese wean their babies onto a mushy rice called congee and as Leach (1989) points out, in California and Israel avocado pears are a common weaning food. What is important is that they are pure foods with no added sugar, salt or 'E' number additives. New tastes should be introduced slowly, giving the baby one new food at a time. Food needs to be mushy (puréed through a sieve) or liquidized, as the baby will not have teeth to chew lumps. The food needs to be of such a consistency that the baby can suck it from the spoon.

When introducing the baby to solid foods it is usual to decide on one feed, i.e. lunchtime or early evening feed, as the regular time when solids will be introduced. They can be given before or after the milk feed, although some practitioners believe that the baby may be more interested in the solid food if it is given before the milk feed. The baby can be fed whilst being held on the lap of the carer or can be sat in a high (or low) chair. A sterilized plastic teaspoon is used to give the baby the food. Make sure that babies have a bib or other protection for their clothes as they are inclined to spit the food out or let the food dribble out of their mouths. One or two teaspoons of food are quite adequate in the first instance. Once you have discovered which foods the baby likes then the quantity can be increased. If the baby does not like the taste of a particular food do not force it to eat; the food can be reintroduced at a later date when the child has got used to a wider variety of foods.

Around 6 months of age the baby will start to chew, although it will have no teeth at this stage. During the next 3 months the baby is able to move from puréed food to food with lumps. This is a good time to introduce finger foods such as a piece of carrot, a crust of bread or a rusk. Never leave a baby alone with finger foods as it could break off a chunk of food and this could choke it. When large chunks do break off it is safest to remove these from the baby.

As babies become more involved with the process of eating solid food so they will want to feed themselves. This is a good time to give them a spoon of their own and they can start to learn to feed themselves. Between the ages of 5 and 8 months the baby will learn to drink from a cup (or feeder cup) and this will cut out the necessity for bottle or breast feeds. As the baby eats a larger variety and larger amounts of solid food, so the intake of milk feeds can be cut down. By the end of the first year the baby may only be having a milk feed before going to bed in the evening. Sucking is a comforting and pleasurable experience for babies and they may be resistant to losing this altogether.

Mealtimes should be a happy, pleasant experience for babies and plenty of time should be given to enable them to learn to feed by themselves. However, this can also be a very messy process, so their clothes and the area around the high chair need to be well protected.

CARE OF BABIES

Nappy Changing

In most Western countries, mothers will have a choice of which type of nappy she will use on her baby. There is a wide choice of disposable nappies available on the market which includes nappies designed to fit the size and gender of the baby. Disposable nappies can be expensive, but in calculating the expense a mother needs to take into consideration the cost of washing and drying terry towelling nappies. There is a wide choice in terry towelling nappies that come in different qualities, thicknesses and at differing prices. Some makes of terry towelling nappies come shaped with Velcro fastenings. For families that have modern washing machines there is no problem in dealing with laundering of terry towelling nappies; however, for the family without a washing machine, disposable nappies may be the most practical solution. Some mothers may choose to use towelling nappies for most of the time and only use disposable nappies when they take the baby away from home. Mothers who know that they intend to have a large family may opt for high quality terry towelling nappies as these will last through a number of children. The decision about which type of nappy to choose will depend upon the mother's preference and her domestic situation. A baby will need to be changed on average about six times a day, so in one week a baby will need about 50 disposable nappies or alternatively two dozen terry towelling nappies (to allow for washing and drying between use). A baby should not be left in a soiled or wet nappy for lengthy periods of time as this will not only be uncomfortable but will cause nappy rash.

Using terry towelling nappies

Terry towelling nappies need to be cleaned, sterilized and washed in boiling water between each usage. They also need to be thoroughly dried and aired before they are reused. On removal, a soiled or wet terry towelling nappy first needs to be sluiced in a bucket of cold water, then rinsed and placed in a lidded bucket containing water and a chemical sterilizing agent such as Napisan. The nappy is left in the sterilizing solution for the period of time recommended in the manufacturer's instructions. Once they have been sterilized nappies can be washed in a washing machine using the hottest cycle. Non-biological washing powder must be used, as any other type of powder is likely to cause rashes or allergies to the baby's skin. Nappies must always be thoroughly rinsed using the full rinse cycle on the machine. Adding a fabric conditioner which is suitable for sensitive skins to the rinse cycle will keep the nappies fluffy and soft.

There are a number of ways of folding terry towelling nappies so that they fit the baby properly and offer the fullest amount of protection in the right places (see diagram on page 122). Only safety nappy pins must be used to secure the nappy as these have a special mechanism that prevents them from coming open by themselves. If terry towelling nappies are used then plastic pants will need to be put over the nappy to prevent bedding and clothing getting soiled. Wherever possible it is better for the baby's skin if plastic pants can be left off for periods of time (particularly during the night) to let the air circulate around the nappy and help the prevention of nappy rash. Plastic pants will need to be sterilized and washed in the same way as nappies.

Changing a nappy

In the home or the nursery there should be a specific area where the baby is changed. In this area there needs to be a trolley or shelf which contains all the things needed to change a baby: buckets or bins in which to place the soiled nappies, access to hot and cold water and a table or shelf which is large enough to accommodate a baby changing mat. If there is not a changing area available then before changing the baby it will be necessary to gather together all the things that you will need, for example:

- Changing mat
- Warm water in a bowl
- Cotton wool balls or baby wet wipes
- Barrier cream such as zinc and castor oil
- Toilet roll or tissues
- Clean nappy (if terry towelling you will also need plastic pants)
- Container for the soiled nappy.

Before changing the baby you should wash your hands and put on the appropriate protective clothing, i.e. disposable plastic apron. Lie the baby on the changing mat and undo or remove any clothing in order to get access to the nappy. *Remember, a baby must never, ever be left alone on a changing mat that is above floor level.*

Undo the nappy fastening, hold the baby's ankles together and lift the baby's bottom, remove the nappy and place in a bucket or other receptacle. Clean any faecal material with toilet roll. Using moist cotton wool or baby wipe, clean the genital area first and then clean backwards towards the buttocks. Make sure that all faecal material or urine is removed. Dry the area thoroughly and apply the barrier cream. Put on the clean nappy and secure it. Put the baby in a safe place and then wash your hands.

Babies will usually need changing following a feed and this should be part of the routine care. They will also need checking at other regular intervals during the day to ensure that they do not have a wet or soiled nappy. Some babies do not like lying in a soiled or wet nappy and will let you know about this by crying until they are changed.

Nappy rash (see Chapter 2)

A common cause of nappy rash in the first month of life is thrush. This is an infection caused by a fungus, which lives in warm moist areas such as mouth, intestines or vagina. It is common for newborn babies to become infected with this from the mother's birth canal. An anti-fungal cream from the doctor easily treats it.

Bathing a Baby

In most situations, babies are bathed using a baby bath; however, a baby can be bathed in a large bowl or in a large sink. The baby bath should be on a purpose-made stand or placed on a secure table or other flat surface. There are baby baths which fit into the adult bath or across the top of the adult bath. Whatever receptacle is used for bathing the baby, it is important that it is on a secure surface where it cannot tip over and in a position that is easily reached by the person carrying out the bathing. Before bathing the baby all the equipment

Two ways of folding a terry towelling nappy.

1. Fold the nappy in half to make a triangle.

2. Lay the baby on the nappy with his waist on the widest part. Then bring up one corner between his legs.

3. Fold the sides over to the middle and hold with one hand.

4. Secure the nappy with a safety pin.

1. Fold the nappy into a kite shape.

2. Lay the baby on the nappy at the level of his waistline.

3. Fold a side corner over and bring the bottom flap up between his legs. Pin to the side corner.

4. Do the same with the other side corner. Tuck it under the front flap, and secure with a safety pin at the corner.

that will be needed should be placed within easy reach of the bath. All toiletries such as soap, talcum powder, shampoo, skin lotions and creams should be of a type that is suitable for babies or sensitive skin. There are a large number of these products on the market and they are all hypoallergenic and so suitable for use on baby skin. In addition to the above items you will also need a small bowl of boiled water that has been left to cool, cotton wool balls, clean nappy, clean clothes, a warm towel, and a bucket for the soiled nappy and dirty clothes. Once all these items have been gathered together, fill the bath two-thirds full of warm water (remembering to put the cold water in first). Test the temperature of the water by dipping your elbow into the water; it should be comfortably warm but not hot.

It is important during the whole process of bathing that the baby is held firmly so that it feels secure. The baby should be undressed on a changing mat or on your lap lying on a towel. Remove all the baby's clothes except the nappy and wrap the baby in the warm towel. Wash the baby's face with cotton wool moistened in the cooled boiled water. With moist cotton wool clean the area around the eyes using a clean piece of cotton wool for each eye. Holding the baby securely, hold its head over the bath and with your free hand wet the head, shampoo the scalp and then rinse away all traces of soap and dry with a towel. Do not be afraid to wash the fontanelle (soft spot) on top of the baby's head. Remove the baby's

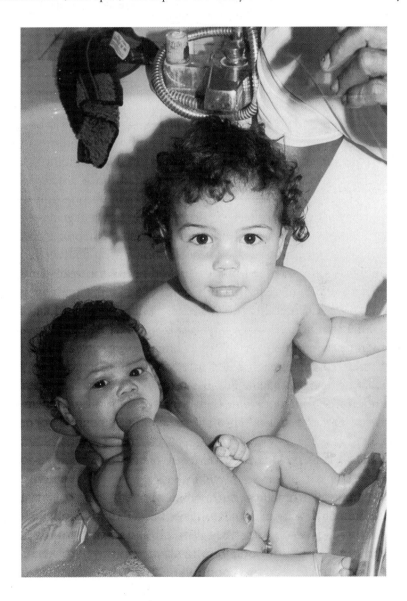

nappy; clean the bottom with damp cotton wool. Lower the baby into the bath whilst keeping your arm securely around it for support. Never let go of the baby when it is in the bath. Wash the baby thoroughly whilst giving it time to kick and splash in the water. Talk to the baby while you are bathing it, as bath time should be an enjoyable experience in which the whole family can participate. Lift the baby out of the bath and wrap it in a warm towel. Pat the baby dry and apply any necessary creams or lotions. Put on a clean nappy, clean clothes and place the baby somewhere safe whilst you tidy away the bath equipment.

A note of caution: many child care workers do not get the opportunity to bath a baby and may learn by simulation using a replica such as a life size doll; however, a soapy, moving real life baby is not always easy to control. If, on completing your training, you are in employment where you need to bath a baby and have not done this before, you must tell your employers so that they can supervise you in this task until you are competent and confident.

Reducing the Risk of Cot Death

Cot death or sudden infant death syndrome (SIDS) is the term used to describe a baby who dies from no identifiable cause. In the UK it is the commonest cause of death in children under 1 year of age, the highest figures being in children aged under 6 months old. Recent research has shown that there are precautions which can be taken to reduce the risk of cot death. Sadly, there is no advice which will guarantee that a baby will not die, but taking the precautions will lessen the risk. The Foundation for the Study of Infant Deaths advises the following:

- Place the baby on the back to sleep.
- Don't smoke and avoid placing the baby in smoky atmospheres.
- Do not let the baby get too hot.
- Keep the baby's head uncovered.
- Place the baby in the cot with its feet at the foot of the cot or pram (this is referred to as the 'feet to foot' position).
- If you think the baby is unwell contact the doctor.

Babies who are exposed to tobacco smoke in the air they breathe are also at greater risk of cot death. It is also advised that mothers and fathers give up smoking during the pregnancy period.

Babies do not need hot rooms. The ideal room temperature is 18°C (65°F). Babies lose excess heat from their heads so when putting them to bed do not cover their heads with bedclothes, hoods, hats etc. When bringing a baby from the outdoors into a warm room remember to remove the extra clothing as soon as you come inside. Duvets should not be used as bedclothes for babies under 1 year of age and bedclothes should be made of natural fibres, preferably cotton. Babies should never sleep with a hot water bottle or electric blanket, next to a radiator, heater or fire, or in direct sunshine.

It is also recommended that a cot is made up so that babies sleep 'feet to foot'; in other words, the baby's feet are at the foot of the cot and the blankets only cover the length of the baby. This reduces the risk of the baby getting its head under the blankets and being unable to regulate heat loss through the head. Parents and carers are advised to watch the press for any updated advice on the precautions relating to cot death as research into the subject is constantly being undertaken. As a result of the most recent research findings the above advice is the latest being publicized by the Foundation for the Study of Infant Deaths (FSID) (this is the most current at the time of going to press); however, this may alter as new research findings are published. It is useful to check with the Foundation periodically to get the most up to date information (the address is in the Appendix at the back of this book). The Foundation has also developed a scheme to provide support for families who have had a child die through cot death. The scheme is called Care of the Next Infant (CONI) and involves such services as additional visits by the Health Visitor, an apnoea alarm to monitor the baby's breathing and additional support from the GP.

Sleep Patterns of Babies

Not all babies will develop the same sleep patterns but most will settle into some type of routine during the first month. During the first year, babies are likely to sleep on average 14–16 hours per day. Half the sleeping time will be during the night and the remainder during the day. When babies sleep they divide the sleeping time into blocks of 2–3 hours with a wakeful period in between each block. As Kakar (1981) points out, putting children down to sleep at a regular time is a very 'western' idea. In Indian culture a child will 'sleep when it sleeps, wake up when it wakes up'. However, when parents work and where there is no extended family to help out, it is easier to get the child into a sleep routine that fits in with the routine of the parents and this can be achieved by putting children down to sleep at regular intervals during the day.

In order to promote sleep the baby needs to be in a comfortable environment, wearing comfortable clothes, not overwrapped or too hot, preferably recently fed and changed. Babies should be put somewhere quiet to sleep as loud noises will waken them.

Sleep and rest are necessary to promote the functioning of the circulatory and respiratory systems, to give the brain and nervous system a chance to rest, to prevent fretfulness and irritability, and generally to help the rebuilding of energy in the body.

Stimulating Babies

All babies need stimulation in order to develop intellectually, physically, socially, emotionally and linguistically. Babies develop at their own pace, and the rate of development may be dependent upon the amount and type of stimulation they are given. Different families and different lifestyles will offer different types of stimulation: for example, a baby carried in a sling will have a very different view of the world than a baby who is in a pram; babies in hot climates are able to benefit from an outdoor lifestyle which offers them a very different experience of movement and space compared with babies who grow up in high rise flats. Developmental scales and charts must therefore be used only as a guide and never viewed as 'tablets of stone' as it is unlikely that there is any baby who develops at a rate 'according to the charts'.

Jean Piaget in 1953 described the early stages of children's cognitive development as the sensorimotor period. This is a very apt description, as this is the period when children learn through use of their senses and fine and gross motor movements (Bee 1992). Evans (1978) writing about the HighScope system describes the first year of life in a different way:

- the heads up stage (0–1 month)
- the looker stage (1–4 months)
- the creeper crawler stage (4–8 months)
- the walker stage (8–12 months).

The ages are approximate as each child will grow at its own rate and some traits will stand out more than others.

There are numerous books available on child development which go into each stage in great detail. In the confines of this chapter it is only possible to take a cursory look at development and this has been done specifically in relation to examples of some of the ways in which babies can be stimulated during the first year of life. Opportunities to stimulate babies should not be lost or overlooked. The daily routine offers times when there is a one-to-one relationship between the child and the adult, for example changing, bathing, feeding and dressing; all of these times offer good opportunities for the adult to talk to the baby and play with the baby. Babies will soon come to recognize the voices of the different adults

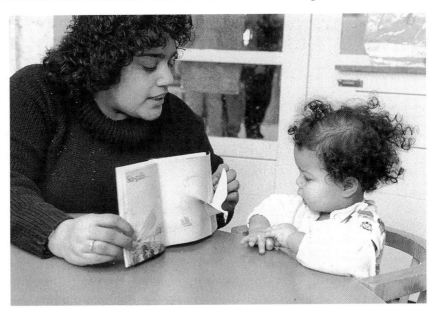

who care for them. At around 1–2 months the baby will respond to the sound of the adult's voice by trying to communicate with cooing and repeated vowel sounds.

It is not necessary to buy lots of toys in order to stimulate the baby. Mobiles, stuffed toys, balls etc. can be homemade or, at a later stage in their development, wooden spoons, saucepans and empty cardboard boxes all provide useful items for babies to explore. However, it is important to ensure that any commercially bought toys have the British Standard Safety Kitemark or the lion mark and are labelled as being safe to use with children aged 1 year and under.

In the first 3 months of life babies learn through their senses (sight, hearing, taste, touch, smell), therefore it is a good idea to provide stimulation through these senses. A mobile placed above the cot at a distance of 20–25 cm (8 inches) from the child's eyes will help the baby focus. If the mobile also has a noise, such as a bell, it will also stimulate the baby's hearing and offer an added interest. Between 2 and 4 months the baby will smile in response to a familiar face. The baby will be able to raise its head, reach for objects and be able to clasp and unclasp its hands. At this stage, in addition to the mobile, a rattle is useful as this can be placed in the baby's hands. Babies will like objects of different colours and textures, and a baby mirror fixed at eye level outside the cot will attract their attention when they turn their heads towards it. Babies at this stage of development do not have what psychologists refer to as 'object permanence'. This means that when the toy has gone from the baby's view the baby does not look for or reach for the toy but just forgets it. When the baby drops the rattle it is forgotten; as the old adage says, 'out of sight out of mind'.

Between 4 and 6 months babies should have good back and head control and be able to sit up. Around this time they develop the ability to pick up objects. They will now need more space and encouragement to move about and this can be done by placing bright colourful objects near to them that they can reach out for and grasp. This is the time they like to sit or lie on a blanket on the floor and play with toys such as a rattle, brightly coloured soft balls and things that can be grasped and investigated such as textured balls, small cardboard boxes etc. It is to be remembered that at this stage babies use their mouths to explore objects, so all toys must be checked for safety. At this stage babies are also exploring their own bodies and they like moving their arms and legs, particularly if this movement can also move a mobile or a rattle which will produce a sound. Bath time is also good fun and babies will quickly learn to kick and splash about in the water. Between 6 and 8 months the baby will be able to sit alone, turn towards sound and be able to transfer objects from hand to hand. It is around this time that babies begin to develop object permanence. When they drop a toy from their high chair or cot they will look over the edge to see where it has gone. Many children find this dropping of objects a very enjoyable game when there is an adult present to pick them up! At this stage they are beginning to explore the world around them so they will need plenty of space to move around. Balls, stacking or nesting toys, large bricks and blocks are very useful for developing movement and enabling the baby to learn about space. At this stage babies will start to enjoy nursery rhymes that are active and repetitive, for example 'Incy Wincy Spider', 'Round and Round the Garden' and 'Pat-a-Cake'. They will babble using consonants and vowel sounds, trying out new sound patterns. They will have good hand to mouth coordination and will use the mouth to explore objects and even furniture.

Around 8–10 months babies will reach the crawling/creeping stage and will try to pull themselves into a standing position. It is the time when special care needs to be taken to make sure that they are in a safe environment; particular attention should be paid to furniture as this needs to be stable and the corners of tables and chairs covered with soft protectors (these can be obtained from baby supply shops such as Mothercare). At this stage they will like to play games such as 'peek-a-boo' and games where they are shown a favourite object which is hidden from their sight and then revealed. Brightly coloured simple picture books will also be attractive to them, particularly those that contain familiar objects that can be named by the adult and the baby then has the opportunity to try to say the word. At this stage they will enjoy playing with household implements such as saucepans, wooden spoons, measuring spoons, a plastic jug etc.

At around 10–12 months they will probably be able to stand by themselves, will be able to use a spoon and can say their first words. This is also the time when they are exploring everything around them and extra safety precautions need to be taken; safety locks on cupboards, refrigerators and freezers, and gates on kitchen doors and at the foot of stairs all help to cut down the risks of accidents. A sturdy babywalker or push-along toy will encourage them to take their first steps whilst still being able to hold on for support. They will soon learn to push the walker towards a toy or other object that they are trying to reach. Activity centres, musical instruments such as xylophones or shakers, bells, building materials such as wooden bricks, and cardboard boxes (particularly very large ones which they can crawl inside) help develop the child's skills whilst making it fun to learn.

Elinor Goldschmied is the pioneer of the 'treasure basket' and 'heuristic play' for under-2-year-olds. The word heuristic comes from the Greek word *eurisko* which means 'to discover or reach an understanding of'. Heuristic play is provided by enabling babies to explore natural objects through the medium of a treasure basket. The treasure basket is a bag or basket containing a number of every-day natural objects that the child can explore and in doing so dis-cover the properties of these objects. For heuristic play there is a need to have the same object in different sizes, objects which stack, objects of different colours and weights. For the under-1-year-olds, who will be finding out the very basic attributes of simple objects, a treasure basket containing a number of different objects is suffi-cient. The types of objects that can go in a treasure basket are as follows:

Natural objects:
Fir cones, shells, big feathers, corks, avocado pear stone, pumice stone etc.

Objects of natural materials:
Woollen ball, small shoe brush, bone ring, shaving brush, small raffia mat etc.

Wooden objects:
Small boxes, castanets, napkin ring, clothes pegs, egg cup, cotton reel etc.

Metal objects:
Spoons, bunch of keys, tea strainer, metal beaker, small tins, bunch of bells, bicycle bell etc.

Objects in leather, textile, rubber, fur:
Small teddy bear, fur ball, leather purse, velvet powder puff, coloured marble eggs, bath plug and chain, etc.

Paper and cardboard objects:
Greaseproof paper, tinfoil, small cardboard boxes etc.

(Goldschmied 1989)

The main purpose of the objects in the treasure basket is to offer stimulus to the child's senses, and Goldschmied states that it is for this reason that plastic items are not included in the objects as they have little stimulus to offer. It must not be forgotten that any objects in a treasure basket are likely to be put into the child's mouth so they must not be small enough for the child to swallow or danger-ous in design or toxic. Children can then put their hands in the basket and each object will teach them something about shape, size, colour, hardness, softness and texture (rough, smooth etc.). Offering smaller baskets will enable the child to manipulate the objects and move them from place to place. The adult has the role of facilitator by collecting the objects together and making them available to the child. When the child is playing the adult can observe what the child does and which objects interest the child most. Even very young children will spend long periods of concentration playing with the objects in a treasure basket.

Key Worker System

Research has shown (particularly that done by John Bowlby and James and Elizabeth Robertson (Bowlby 1971, 1975)) that when babies are in day care and are handled by a number of people they can become disturbed as they are unable to bond with one person. The idea of a key worker system is that only one or two people are assigned to look after a particular baby. In this way the baby is able to develop a relationship with the key workers assigned to it. The key workers are also able to gain the confidence of the parent or primary carer as part of the shared care. A key worker system is good practice when dealing with all children but particularly with children aged under 18 months. However, there have been some objections to the system from both staff and nursery managers. Staff often feel that all children should be treated equally and the key worker system gives some children more attention than others; the managers have difficulty in staffing all sections of the nursery if certain members of staff are assigned to care for particular children.

Parental Involvement

It is important that the child care worker responsible for the baby works with the parents or primary carer so that the child has the best possible care; shared care is the best practice. Many parents lack confidence in dealing with their child, particularly if it is a first baby, and will be looking for reassurance from the childminder or child care worker. Ante-natal classes which concentrate on parent education would have given the parents some ideas as to how the baby will develop in the first few months of life. In the early days the midwife and health visitor will be available to advise and instruct. If a mother is lacking in confidence it is very useful to be able to put her in touch with other mothers. Organizations such as PIPPIN (Parent Infant Project) and Meet-a-Mum provide a networking system between mothers with local group meetings and problem-solving skills for new parents (addresses in Appendix).

It is important that when the parents develop a new skill they are encouraged and praised by the child care worker. It is very easy for the child care worker to take over completely and make the parents feel useless and de-skilled. The parents have to cope in the evenings and at weekends and it is important for the continuity of the child's care for the parents to know exactly how to handle their child in the very numerous situations that may arise. If the child care worker learns a new technique which encourages the child to do something better then this should be shared with the parents; likewise, if the child reaches a particular developmental stage when it is with the child care worker then the parents need to be informed that the baby can now drink from a cup, sit up, roll over etc.

ASSIGNMENTS

1. Describe how you would prepare a bottle feed for a 2-month-old baby.

2. 'Breast milk is best.' Discuss this statement.

3. Describe the procedure for changing a baby's nappy.

4. What is 'sudden infant death syndrome' and what precautions can be taken to lower the risk of this happening?

5. Describe how you would bath a 6-month-old baby.

6. What is heuristic play? What type of activities could you offer to a 1 year old to develop this type of play?

7. What do you understand by the term 'shared care'? Why is it important to promote 'shared care'?

PRACTICAL ACTIVITIES

1. Make a series of observations of children at 2 months, 6 months, 8 months and 1 year from the point of view of the following developmental areas: physical, language, intellectual and emotional.

2. Make a Treasure Basket for a baby of 8 months of age then observe what the child does with this. Write up your observation and add your own evaluation.

3. Write the menus for a week for an 8-month-old baby who is partially weaned and only has a bottle feed before going to bed at night.

4. Arrange an outing for a baby of 9 months old explaining why you have chosen the place to visit and what the baby will learn from the visit.

References

Bee H 1992 The developing child, 6th edn. Harper Collins, New York

Bowlby J 1953 Child care and the growth of love. Pelican, London

Bowlby J 1971 Attachment and loss, Vol 1. Penguin, London

Bowlby J 1975 Attachment and loss, Vol 2. Penguin, London

Evans J 1978 Good beginnings. HighScope Press, Ypsilanti, USA

Goldschmied E 1989 Play and learning in the first year of life. In: Williams V (ed) Babies in daycare: an examination of the issues. The Daycare Trust, London

Kakar S 1981 The inner world – a psychoanalytic study of children and society in India. Oxford University Press, Delhi

Leach P 1989 Baby and child: from birth to age five. Penguin, London

Reid J 1995 More than meets the eye. New research into babies. Nursery World 23 November:12

Further reading

■ Abbott L, Moylett H (eds) 1997 Working with the under 3's: responding to children's needs. Open University Press, Buckingham

■ Bowlby J 1979 The making and breaking of affectional bonds. Tavistock, London

■ Cowley L 1994 Young children in group day care: guidelines for good practice, 2nd edn. National Children's Bureau, London

■ Goldschmied E 1987 Infants at work (notes). National Children's Bureau, London

■ Goldschmied E 1990 What to do with under twos. Heuristic play. Infants learning. In: Babies and toddlers: carers and educators. Quality for the under threes. National Children's Bureau, London

■ Goldschmied E, Jackson S 1997 People under three: young children in day care. Routledge, London

■ Hilton T, Messenger M 1993 The Great Ormond Street book of baby and child care. Bodley Head, London

■ Jolly H 1986 Book of child care. Unwin Paperbacks, London

■ Leach P 1997 Your baby and child: essential guide for every parent. Penguin, London

■ Pugh G, De'Ath E, Smith C 1994 Confident parents, confident children. National Children's Bureau, London

■ Sheridan MD (revised and updated by Frost M, Sharma A) 1997 From birth to five years: children's developmental progress. Routledge, London

■ Vincent Priya J 1992 Birth traditions and modern pregnancy care. Element, Dorset

■ Williams V (ed) 1989 Babies in daycare: an examination of the issues. The Daycare Trust, London

Chapter 6

Child Development

This chapter covers underpinning knowledge for all NVQs or courses in Early Years Care and Education, including the CACHE Diploma and Certificate. Whilst it is not linked with specific units or modules the material in this chapter underpins all work with children.

INTRODUCTION

Child development is the study of how children develop as they grow physically, intellectually, linguistically, emotionally and socially (the well-known mnemonic (memory aid) for this being PILES. In some books intellectual development is described as cognitive development. Whilst all human beings follow the same developmental pattern or order of development, there is great variety in individual performance. In other words children develop at different rates according to their environment, their abilities, the stimulation they receive and the opportunities that they are given to learn new skills. An understanding of child development is a very important part of the underpinning knowledge required by parents and child care workers. Having a knowledge of child development enables parents and carers to offer children the relevant experiences in order to aid their developmental progress.

The development of children is dependent upon a number of factors; however, the academics and researchers who produce theories on child development are often specialists in only one field and therefore study one area of development in depth. A study undertaken in this way may be in isolation from the other factors that are involved. Taken at its most literal, a knowledge of child development can be a very dangerous tool if it is used without thought or reference to all the factors which may have an effect upon it. It is important always to look at the child as a whole (the holistic view) and to take into consideration social and cultural factors.

For convenience, child development is described in a form that detracts from the holistic view of the child. It must therefore be remembered that each aspect of development is like a piece of a jigsaw puzzle which may be interesting in itself but only makes sense when it is part of the whole picture. For example children who are feeling unwell (physical) will not want to participate in learning activities or play (intellectual), they may be fretful and irritable (emotional) and may not respond to attempts to include them in interaction with their parents or carers or others (social), and they may revert to baby talk to explain their symptoms (linguistic).

A good method of studying child development is by observing children and this is why most child care courses place a great emphasis on child observations. Many students begin to learn the skill of observing by watching videos of children in different stages of development; following this they progress to carrying out observations when they are in practical work placements. With a knowledge of child development theories a student can then evaluate the observation. There are a large number of books devoted just to child development and some of these can be found in the reference section at the end of this chapter. Suffice to say that it is impossible to give more than a brief outline of development within the confines of this chapter. It needs to be remembered that there is not one single child development theorist who is accepted by all the experts; most people use ideas from a number of theorists.

In describing aspects of child development, writers use terms such as 'norm', 'milestones', 'approximate ages', 'stages' etc. In order to produce a set of benchmarks along the development continuum. It is necessary for writers to do this in order to transfer ideas and theories in a way that can be understood by their readers. All children develop at their own pace and there is unlikely to be in existence a 'normal' child who reaches all the milestones at the target ages as laid down in the literature.

CULTURAL ASPECTS OF CHILD DEVELOPMENT

Cassie Landers (1995) describes culture as 'a body of learned meaning and shared information transmitted from generation to generation through interaction … therefore cultural variations in child rearing influence children's mental, emotional and social development, just as such variations determine which language a child will eventually speak. Parental approaches to child-rearing in different cultures are similar in some ways but different in others.'

This broad definition of culture put forward by Landers (1995) enables those involved with child development to take culture into account in its widest sense. In other words, culture encompasses class, race, ethnicity, environment, religion, politics, gender, and anything else that may contribute towards the way in which a family group forms its value system. It is these values which are then passed on from generation to generation. Such values will influence the way parents and carers approach child rearing and view child development. For example, environmental issues such as climate will influence the culture. Hot countries have an outdoor culture, whereas cold and temperate countries will have an indoor culture. Children living in hot countries are likely to have more freedom in terms of space and this in turn may lead to them having earlier developmental patterns in gross motor movements such as walking, running, jumping, climbing etc.

Families and individuals are able to accept or reject these shared values which are continually being updated and refashioned. When studying child development it needs to be remembered that parents will interpret the world to the child and this interpretation will be influenced by how the adults see the world (cultural influences). It is also necessary for child care workers to consider how their own value systems and culture influence the ways in which they deal with children and their parents.

More recently people have begun to take an interest in children's spiritual development and this is an area which features in the Desirable Learning Goals devised by the Qualifications and Curriculum Authority 1999. Spiritual development must not be confused with religious development. Spiritual development concerns a child's sense of awe, wonder, knowing what is good and what is bad, relating to other children and adults, knowing what makes them happy, what may hurt them and what makes them sad. As children get older (8+ years) these concepts become more abstract and develop into what could be considered as the child's moral development: a sense of justice/injustice, good versus evil, understanding of right and wrong etc.

CHILD DEVELOPMENT THEORISTS

As already stated there is not one theorist who satisfies all the experts in the field; however, it might be useful to have some knowledge of the most well known. It is to be noted that the following are the author's choice in terms of importance but there are many other theorists who are not mentioned here and whose work may have an impact on the interpretation of children's development.

Piaget, Jean (1896–1980)

This Swiss biologist and psychologist is a central figure in the school of cognitive development theory. Piaget's theories, which were based upon many years of research and observation of children, outlined stages of intellectual development (see Table 6.1).

Piaget's work shows that children go through stages in learning and before a child can progress from one stage to another, both maturation (internal growth) and appropriate learning must take place. Special training to try to enhance/speed up this process is only temporarily effective and children tend to revert to their natural developmental level. Piaget showed that intellectual development is not simply an accumulation of changes but is a process whereby children construct their own understanding of self, others and the world around them. In order to do this children are consistently trying to adapt to the world around them, which leads them to pass through stages of

Table 6.1 *Piaget's stages of intellectual development*

Stage	Approximate ages
1. *Sensorimotor period*	Birth to 2 years
Sub-stage I	Birth to 1 month
Sub-stage II	1–4 months
Sub-stage III	4–10 months
Sub-stage IV	10–12 months
Sub-stage V	12–18 months
Sub-stage VI	18 months to 2 years
2. *Pre-operational thought period*	2–7 years
Preconceptual phase	2–4 years
Intuitive phase	4–7 years
3. *Period of concrete operations*	7–11 years
4. *Period of formal operations*	11–15 years

increasing complexity of thought. Piaget called these stages sensorimotor, pre-operational thought, concrete operations and formal operations. Piaget states that there is a constant interaction between emotional and intellectual aspects of development so that in times of stress a child may regress to an earlier level of thinking. Emotional difficulties can prevent progression to the next level of thinking and may render the person unable ever to reach full logical functioning.

There has been criticism of Piaget's theories on the grounds that he seems to have been wrong about the way in which cognitive skills develop. Work by Susan Martorano (1977) has shown that a child may perform at one stage on one task and at another stage on a second task even though the two tasks seem to require the same basic cognitive thought.

Freud, Sigmund (1856–1939)

Freud was the founder of a school of thought known as psychoanalysis that states that the development of the child's personality is greatly influenced by the child's relationship with its parents. According to Freud the infant's relationship with its mother develops as a secondary consequence of the way she provides relief from hunger and thirst. The child develops emotional dependence upon the mother by its own efforts to reduce the discomfort of hunger and thirst. Freud maintained that the child's developmental progress could be seen in psychosexual stages (see Table 6.2). The stages are characterized by certain sources of sexual gratification.

Erikson, Erik (1902–1994)

The psychologist Erikson looked primarily at social development of children. Erikson worked with Freud's daughter Anna who concentrated most of her work on children, particularly children who had

Table 6.2 *Freud's stages of psychosexual development*

Stage	Approximate age	Characteristics
Oral	0–8 months	Sources of pleasure include sucking, biting, swallowing, playing with lips; preoccupation with immediate gratification of impulses
Anal	8–18 months	Sources of sexual gratification include expelling faeces and urinating, as well as retaining faeces
Phallic	18 months to 6 years	Child becomes concerned with genitals; source of sexual pleasure involves manipulating genitals; period of Oedipus or Electra complex
Latency	6–11 years	Loss of interest in sexual gratification; identification with same-sexed parent

survived the Nazi concentration camps. Erikson's theory puts forward eight developmental stages (the first four are described in Table 6.3). Erikson's stages of development cover the whole life-span, not just the period of childhood.

The eight stages are as follows:

1. Basic trust versus basic mistrust
2. Autonomy versus shame, doubt
3. Initiative versus guilt
4. Industry versus inferiority
5. Identity versus role confusion

Table 6.3 *Erikson's development phases, 0–9 years*

Approximate ages	Psychosocial crises	Radius of significant relations	Psychosocial modalities	Psychosexual stages
0–8 months	1. Trust versus mistrust	Maternal person	To get: to give in and return	Oral–respiratory sensory–kinesthetic
8–18 months	2. Autonomy versus shame and doubt	Parental persons	To hold on: to let go	Anal–urethral, muscular– (retentive–eliminative)
18 months to 6 years	3. Initiative versus guilt	Basic family	To make (going after): to make like (playing)	Infantile–genital locomotor
6–9 years	4. Industry versus inferiority	Neighbourhood, school	To make things (completing): to make things together	Latency

6. Intimacy versus isolation
7. Generativity versus stagnation
8. Ego integrity versus despair.

Erikson's theory argues that the presence of conflict stemming from the person's need to adapt to a social environment produces certain types of thinking. Resolution of the conflict results in the development of a new competence. Erikson sees the first characteristic of infancy as 'trust versus mistrust', i.e. a natural mistrust of the world about which the child knows nothing and yet an accompanying need to arrive at feelings of security and trust. Although confrontation and resolution of this and other conflicts continues throughout life, the safe and reliable environment provided for the child helps him to overcome the early mistrust. As does Freud, Erikson believes that the basic mistrust centres around bodily functions such as eating and emotions associated with these functions.

The differences between Freud and Erikson are that Freud maintains that all the cognitive skills develop only because the child needs them to obtain gratification whereas Erikson maintains that the ego functions are presumed to develop independently even though they are used to obtain basic gratification. For a fuller explanation of these theories see Bee (1992, Ch. 7).

Bandura, Albert (Born 1925)

Bandura is a social learning theorist who looks primarily at the reinforcement patterns in the environment as being responsible for the differences in children's behaviour patterns. Whilst accepting biological factors such as hormones and inherited characteristics do have a role to play in forming a child's behaviour pattern, Bandura maintains that the greatest influences are the environmental factors. For example, a child care worker who only pays attention to children when they are noisy and rowdy will be reinforcing this type of behaviour pattern and therefore the children will become more rowdy and noisy in order to gain attention. Bandura's theories are the basis for many positive reinforcement programmes that are used with children who exhibit extreme behaviours.

Bruner, Jerome (Born 1915)

Bruner's developmental theories have been influenced by the work of Piaget as they both believe that children are born with a biological organization which enables them to understand the world around them, and as their cognitive structures mature so they can think in an ever more complex way, and that children have an innate curiosity which enables them to explore and adapt to their environment through interaction with it. However, Bruner's theory is not really about stages of development but is three ways of representing the world, enactive, iconic and symbolic, which children develop in that order. Enactive is representation of the world through actions and what has been experienced through a baby's own behaviour. Iconic is when the child builds up a mental image of things it has experienced. Symbolic is the change that occurs around 6–7 years of age and is when language has an influence on thought.

Vygotsky, Lev (1896–1934)

Vygotsky claimed that the most significant moment in the development of the intellect was when speech and practical activity converged. He therefore did not see as separate the way a child developed speech and how the child organized its practical activity. This made Vygotsky a believer in play (the practical activity) going hand in hand with the development of speech. For Vygotsky all speech is about social interaction and communication.

STAGES OF DEVELOPMENT

For other details of development in the first year see Chapter 5.

1–3 Months

Physical development

The newborn baby is endowed with primitive reflex actions, which are responses to stimuli. The earliest and most essential reflex is that of sucking. When placed with their cheek next to the breast babies root around until they find the nipple which they then suck. This is a primitive reflex to satisfy the basic need for food. At 1 month the child begins to associate sucking with satisfaction and comfort and this reflex becomes a voluntary action. Most reflexes disappear within 4 weeks of birth.

At 1 month the baby has lost some of the neonatal reflex actions but will still make reflex walking actions if held standing on a hard surface. If the cheek is touched the baby will turn its head to one side. The baby's head falls forward if it is held in a sitting position to form a C curve with the rest of the body. Grasping, rooting and random movements are present in the first month.

At 3 months the baby shows anticipatory actions by moving arms and legs. The grasp reflex, which is lost by the age of 3 months, is when an adult finger is placed on the palm of each hand and the newborn baby will respond by grasping so tightly that it can be pulled up from the lying position. If a piece of rope is grasped by the baby and suspended above the cot, the baby will hang without danger of falling, such is the strength of the grasping reflex. These early reflexes are seen as precursors to later stages in development such as holding objects and walking. When the baby hears a sudden loud noise it responds with the startle reflex. The arms are flung outwards and then brought in towards the body. Another reflex which is useful is the ability to turn the head to one side when the baby is placed on its back.

Intellectual development

At 1 month of age babies respond to stimuli of light and movement. They turn their heads and eyes towards the light and can follow a pencil light for a little while when it is held about 30 cm (12 inches) away from them. When the light is shone directly at them babies will shut their eyes tight, a defence mechanism which persists through life. If a dangling toy or rattle is shaken about 15–20 cm (6–8 inches) away from the babies' eyes they will follow it as it is moved from side to side. Experiments have shown that babies respond not only to human faces but also to drawings resembling human faces. At 1 month the baby watches the mother's face during feeding.

Feeding presents valuable opportunities for learning and in breast feeding the baby explores taste, smell and touch. It is thought that the senses of touch, taste and smell are more acute at birth. Babies' heightened sensitivity to smell is shown in their ability to distinguish between the smell of breast milk and sugar water.

Helping the child's intellectual development in the first 3 months involves extending the stimulation provided in the everyday activities of feeding, bathing and changing nappies. Babies should be spoken to from birth as this aids development of language and acts as auditory stimulation. Adequate stimulation is essential for all aspects of development; babies left in cots gazing up at white walls and ceilings, deprived of interaction with adults, show all the signs of failing to thrive. In studies undertaken on the long term effects of stimulation in babies it was discovered that babies who had not been stimulated did not learn new tasks as quickly as those who had the right amount of stimulation. However, over-stimulation does not accelerate development; hanging numerous mobiles above a cot, having highly coloured and patterned wallpaper and flowery cot sheets would present over-stimulation and would be likely to cause the baby distress. Thus the right balance needs to be achieved.

A single colourful mobile (which could be home-made) suspended above the cot is sufficient for the first 2–3 months. After this period a more complex shape could be used. Mobiles need to be brightly coloured in order to gain the child's attention. At 1 month the child will simply lie and look at a mobile; at 2 months the child will attempt to hit it, but without success as it has not yet achieved sufficient eye/hand coordination to enable it to make direct contact with the object. Such complex coordination does not develop until around 5 months of age.

Language development

Babbling often begins around 2 months of age and is repeated 'play speech' rather than communication as the baby repeats sounds just for pleasure. Even babies with deaf parents will babble although their parents cannot hear or respond to them. While babbling is not essential to the development of speech it does provide verbal practice which lays the foundation for developing a recognizable language. It is a good idea for the adult to encourage babbling by repeating the sounds that the baby makes. This delights the baby who is encouraged to develop a range of noises.

Emotional development

The formation in early infancy of secure attachments with constant adults is crucial for the child's future emotional development. Security is as much a basic need as food, warmth and protection. A feeling of trust is essential for human relationships. Even at 1 month of age babies respond to a soothing voice and a cuddle. Anxiety or tension can easily be transmitted to the baby through rough handling or a short temper. A mother who is upset and worried and complains that the baby is always crying may not realize how her own emotional distress can upset the baby.

Most mothers tend to position their babies on their left side. This means that the baby can hear the mother's heart beating, and studies show that babies find this very soothing and reminiscent of their intrauterine life. It has also been discovered that babies whose mothers listened to music during pregnancy sleep happily in the first months of life with a radio or record player on.

Social development

While the child's first relationship is usually with its parents, it is also able to form attachments with others, and it is the quality of the interaction (rather than the length) which appears to be the important factor. Whether the primary care-giver is the child's biological mother or not, there will exist from the earliest days a reciprocity of communication. The mother or primary care-giver is sensitive to the baby's signals – smiles, cries or babbling – and her response establishes early socialization as a partnership. The basis for communication is laid in the dialogue between care-giver and baby; the baby responds by imitating or offering another initiative. This important interaction is observed in all the mutual experiences shared by care-giver and baby – feeding, bathing, playing, nappy changing, bedtime – and serves to reinforce and develop the relationship. Thus as the baby learns about its social environment by initiating contact with and responding to its care-giver, the care-giver's interest in the baby increases and so furthers the partnership. At 5 weeks the baby may smile at its care-giver when she talks to the baby and at 6 weeks may 'talk back' by gurgling in response to the care-giver's voice. Observations of babies from birth to 1 month have shown that they will gaze for a longer period of time at the human face or drawings and cut-out images which resemble the face. By 6 weeks, most babies carry out detailed examination of the human face, with the eyes seeming to hold the greatest fascination.

3–6 Months

Physical development

At 3 months of age the baby can keep its head erect for a few seconds when held in the sitting position. This is due to bone and muscle development in the cervical region of the vertebral column; it also enables the baby to move its head to look around. The baby's limbs now move more easily and when placed on its tummy it is able to lift its head and upper trunk using its forearms for support. When the baby is held standing with its feet on a hard surface the

A baby of 6 months can sit upright with support.

legs will sag at the knees. At 3 months the reflex actions have usually disappeared and the baby has some voluntary movements which it likes to repeat. Finger play involves clasping and unclasping hands and the baby likes to watch the movement of its hands. At 5 months the baby can reach out to grasp with both hands. One month later its range of abilities will be extended as it develops the palmar grasp which enables it to use the whole hand as a scoop, and soon the baby will be happy to use just one rather than both hands. At this stage everything is taken to the mouth, as oral exploration is the main sensory activity.

Intellectual development

This stage is characterized by the beginnings of intentional activity in that the baby repeats actions in order to make interesting events last. If small bells are suspended across the cot and the baby discovers the bells will ring if a cord is pulled, it will continue to pull the cord, although not in the sense of using a stimulus to bring about a response as it is not yet old enough to link the activities; the baby simply wants to make an interesting result persist, in the same way that it will repeatedly shake a rattle.

At this stage babies still think that when an object is out of sight it is no longer in existence, and when a toy falls out of their hands it is forgotten if it cannot be seen. At 4–6 months the baby will reach out to take a partially covered object but is unable to obtain an object that has been completely covered by a cloth as the object ceases to exist once it is out of sight. When a 5-month-old baby is presented with a stationary object that proceeds to move, the baby can follow it wherever it goes. The child now seems able to realize that an object can go from place to place through movement, although the child's visual perception (or ability to translate and understand the information it receives through sight) seems to be ahead of its sensorimotor coordination.

Another result of the baby's playing is 'object attainment' which means that it comes to appreciate that an object seen in different ways will still be the same object. Thus when the baby is able to hold the bottle and suck from the teat it will attempt to suck the bottom if the bottle is presented to it upside down. At a later stage, when the baby has come to recognize it is an enduring object, it will turn it round the right way before sucking.

During this period the baby is able to distinguish between simple geometric forms such as circles, squares and triangles. These can be used as mobiles, or plastic shapes can be given to the baby to grasp – provided they are large enough not to be swallowed! Familiarity with three-dimensional shapes can be developed through sight, touch, taste and movement.

Language development

The 6-month-old baby provides a reward for the adult who has constantly persisted with the spoken word as the child vocalizes in single and double syllables which sound very like 'mum' and 'dada', and are eagerly translated as such by delighted parents. Familiar noises like that of the voice of the primary care-giver, preparation of feeds, running water in the bath etc. are greeted with laughs, chuckles and delighted squeals, but screams of annoyance fill the air if the baby's expectations are not fulfilled. The adult cannot ignore these overtures and responds with reinforcement of desired words. The baby quickly realizes that certain sounds provoke a pleased response from the adult and the baby provides its own reinforcement as it shouts to attract attention. The baby also pauses to listen for the response and if it is not forthcoming, shouts again. The baby's powers of imitation are evident as it imitates the coughing, smacking of lips and other sounds that it hears around it.

Emotional development

A firm but gentle way of handling the baby contributes to feelings of security and trust and is particularly necessary for bath time when any hesitation on the adult's part can make the baby scream with terror. At 6 months the baby is clearly able to distinguish between different emotional tones in the voice of the primary care-giver. A quiet but not flat tone of voice, showing interest, care and even delight, will enhance the relationship with the child.

During the first 3 months there are subtle, but no less definite, changes in the relationship between care-giver and child. These changes are partly due to the care-giver's growing self-confidence but also occur in response to the maturational changes in the baby. The baby is now awake more, cries less and spends more time smiling, vocalizing and looking at the care-giver's face. Meanwhile the care-giver is gradually decreasing the amount of very close physical contact, spends more time near the infant, increases affectionate behaviour, provides more stimulation and is more socially responsive towards the child.

Social development

As early as 3 months a baby recognizes the voice of its primary care-giver and shows delight in familiar happenings such as feeding, bathing and dressing, by smiling, cooing and moving its legs and arms. Studies with babies of 4–6 months of age reveal that the younger infants respond happily to multiple images of the care-giver whereas older babies become agitated as they realize that this is unnatural and prefer one stable image. They do not distinguish between strangers and familiars at this stage. Around 6 months, the baby may show anxiety or slight shyness in the presence of strangers – especially if the care-giver is out of sight. The presence of the primary care-giver acts as a pivot on which an enlarging circle of relationships turns. The child gains confidence from the security of firm but gentle handling and the satisfaction of expectations in basic need areas such as feeding.

6–9 Months

Physical development

The baby now holds its head erect with its back straight and although it may be able to sit up alone for a few seconds its back should still be well supported. The baby can raise its head and chest when placed face downwards, and is able to bear its own weight on its feet and bounce up and down when held in the standing position. At this age the baby uses its arm and wrist muscles to pull objects towards it and grasps them with the whole hand using the palmar grasp (eye–hand coordination). The baby has also discovered that its feet are useful playthings and may use them for grasping, although it prefers to put them in its mouth! As the baby is able to sit up with support it will turn its head from side to side and its eyes will follow any movements of objects in its direct vicinity.

At 9 months the child's exploration of its environment involves movement of its trunk in rolling as a preliminary to crawling and standing with support. The child is very observant, manipulates objects by passing them from hand to hand and pokes them with its index finger. The baby can sit alone for up to 15 minutes (on the floor), turn its body sideways and move about by rolling on its tummy. The baby may also begin to crawl, although some children miss out this stage, preferring instead to shuffle along on their bottoms using one hand for support. The baby can stand holding on to a support for a few minutes, but cannot lower itself to the sitting position. When the baby is held standing it takes 'steps' on alternate feet and can stretch out for objects that it sees in front of it. When it picks up items from the floor it uses the finger and thumb in a scissor fashion and is less likely to put objects into its mouth. The child will begin to explore objects by touch or visually or use the object for rhythmic banging.

Intellectual development

If the child is asked to hand over an object it may obey this instruction, but it does not offer objects voluntarily. Object attainment has now extended to a realization of object permanence – the child appreciates that an object, though hidden from sight, still exists and will look under a cloth to find a toy. At this stage children enjoy games of 'peek-a-boo'. This involves temporarily hiding from the baby; providing the play partner reappears fairly soon, the baby can enjoy the game without feeling afraid. Often laughter is mingled with fear, as the child feels insecure when someone leaves it all alone; as yet it cannot appreciate the notion of time or the meaning of temporary. The baby is now able to search in the correct place for the toys it has dropped within reach and will look for toys which have fallen from the pram or chair. The baby's newly developed understanding of object permanence and ability to direct activity towards an end (e.g. removal of a cover before the toy can be discovered) is, according to Piaget, the precursor of adult problem solving.

Bruner uses the term 'early play' to describe the range of activities enjoyed by the 6-month-old after it has learned to hold an object and get it easily to its mouth. 'Mastery play' is what Bruner calls the stage when the baby's actions with the object demonstrate its developing abilities. For example, first the child looks at the object, shakes it, bangs it on the chair, drops it over the edge and before long is able to fit the object into every possible activity. All this newly acquired mastery is applied to every new object, and Bruner found it surprising that at 6–8 months, babies can carry on such varied activities for as long as 30 minutes.

Emotional development

Around 7–8 months of age the child will show a natural anxiety, or 'fear of strangers'. This often upsets members of the wider family circle who are puzzled when the child begins to scream when they approach. However, if the primary carer or another adult who is very close to the child is present the fear can be easily resolved. This 'fear of strangers' combined with the ability to realize that unseen objects still exist (object permanence) explains the delight of the child in playing 'peek-a-boo' type games. Some minor fear can also be exciting. Like adults who love the thrill of fairground rides and enjoy screaming lustily to exhibit this fear, babies scream with delight when a known face suddenly appears from behind a door or bobs up again in front of the pram. However, at this stage, the child will be distressed at any real separation from a familiar person.

Social development

At 9 months the use of hearing and speech in social development is evident as the baby uses babbling noises, loud noises, 'mmm', 'bah bah' and 'duh duh' sounds to attract attention and communicate.

This is highly successful as parents and care-givers eagerly translate these meaningless sounds into 'mummy', 'daddy' and 'baby' and they naturally respond with more attention, reassurance and reinforcement of acceptable behaviour. As previously stated, at this stage the baby may respond negatively to strangers and will not accept them happily unless a familiar adult is present, although it may respond with a 'selective social smile'.

Signs of developmental delay at 5–8 months

Landers (1995) states that a baby who shows any of the following signs of developmental delay should be seen by a doctor or health visitor:

> One or both eyes consistently turns in or out
> Has difficulty getting objects to her mouth
> Does not roll over in either direction by five months
> Does not smile spontaneously by five months
> Cannot sit without help by six months
> Does not smile or make squealing sounds by six months
> Does not actively reach for objects by six or seven months
> Does not bear some weight on legs by six or seven months
> Does not babble by eight months

> (Landers 1995)

9–12 Months

Physical development

From 10–12 months the baby begins to pull itself up to a standing position and can let itself down while holding on to furniture. At 12 months it may try walking around a low table in a sideways fashion. Some babies can stand alone for a few minutes and even walk with one or both hands held by an adult. Other babies may not walk until they are 14–16 months of age, but this is just due to variation in the pace of development. The first movements which indicate that the baby is gaining voluntary control of the small muscles include the pincer grasp, using thumb and index finger, which the baby uses to pick up small toys and small pieces of food. At this stage babies may be experimenting with feeding themselves, but the enormous opportunities for exploratory play with different foods and liquids often take precedence over the necessity to actually eat, although if the child is really hungry the food will eventually find its way into its mouth.

Once they have been shown, babies can click two blocks together or build a tower from two or three small blocks. Whilst most babies at this stage use both hands they may begin to show a preference for one hand; this is the beginning of right and left handedness. The baby can drink from a cup with a little help and can hold a spoon; however, it may have difficulty in using the object properly without help. At this stage the baby is able to clap its hands in imitation of adults and also wave 'bye-bye'.

Exploration of the environment is extended by the baby's ability to crawl, which rapidly leads to standing whilst holding on to furniture, walking with one or both hands held by the adult, or stepping sideways around furniture. The baby's self-confidence increases with its ability to move around.

Intellectual development

Due to the baby's developing ability to coordinate movements it is possible to detect the means and the ends to its activities. The baby may grasp the bell by the handle and ring it in imitation of the adult; it is able to manipulate objects in the environment and will put

(a) Fine motor movements.
(b) Palmar grasp (6 months). (c) Pincer grasp (12 months).
(i) Pointing with index finger (9 months).
(ii) Picking up small objects (12 months).

(a)

(b)

(c)

(i)

(ii)

wooden cubes into a cup or box and then lift them out again. To the baby's delight it may find that it is able to manipulate adults, dropping toys deliberately and watching them fall to the ground, only to be picked up by whoever is passing by and returned to the baby who promptly drops them again! The repetitive action strengthens the child's sense of control over events and demonstrates understanding of 'object permanence' as the child looks in the correct place for the toy which has gone out of sight. Babies at this stage are able to point with their index fingers and as already stated are able to use a pincer movement to pick up small objects. The baby's behaviour indicates that it is able to discriminate between differences in people and things, and it moves from shyness and uneasiness with strangers to an acceptance, although it is still dependent upon its primary carer. Babies are able to begin to understand and perceive relationships between new and old situations and this is helped if the new material has something in common with past experiences. This is the beginning of coming to understand the world around them and the development of concepts that help them to order their understanding of the environment.

Language development

The baby is now able to recognize its own name and turns around in response to its name being called. The baby shows that it is able to understand simple commands accompanied by gestures, such as, 'Give me the spoon', 'Clap your hands'. The baby's self-confidence increases with its knowledge of its own name and the understanding of simple words relating to the world around it e.g. cup, spoon, walk, clap, dinner, ball, car etc. The adult is able to help the baby extend its language by continual repetition and explanation of day-to-day activities.

Emotional development

At this stage babies, as Penelope Leach (1997) points out, have strong emotions but have very little power. Their loves, hates, wishes and desires appear to be as strong as those of adults, but without language and physical mobility they are unable to do anything about them. This in itself leads to frustration and crying in situations which they cannot change. They will also cry at the unexpected, such as changes in routine, changes in the primary carer, going on a swing for the first time, first meeting with a large animal etc. At this stage, apart from hunger or illness, crying is a reaction to fear or an explosion of frustration and anger; some babies may need a comfort object such as a blanket, furry toy or even their thumb.

*Social
development*

As the baby approaches the end of its first year it comes to realize that adults can be used to provide help in play with objects and that objects can be used to gain the attention of adults.

*Signs of
developmental
delay at
12 months*

Landers (1995) states that if babies are exhibiting any of the following signs at 12 months of age then a doctor or health visitor should be consulted:

> Drags one side of the body while crawling (existing for over one month)
> Cannot stand when supported
> Does not search for objects that are hidden while she watches
> Says no single word (such as 'mama' or 'dada')
> Does not learn to use gestures such as waving or shaking the head
> Does not point to objects or pictures
>
> (Landers 1995)

15–18 Months

*Physical
development*

At about 15 months children can usually walk, but unsteadily and there may be frustrations and anger as they bump into furniture. They can also get to their feet alone, sit down backwards (with a bump), or fall forward onto their hands and then sit. They can crawl upstairs and therefore safety measures should include a stair gate, which is strong, stable and able to withstand the child's weight. Leg muscles may be sufficiently developed to enable the child to bend and pick up toys from the floor. The child is able to hold a cup and bring a spoon to its mouth in order to lick it, but may lack sufficient muscle control to hold it in one position for any length of time. At this stage large wheeled toys with handles which are very stable are useful as the child loves to push them and this helps it to practise walking by offering it support. Small muscle control can be seen in the way the child is able to pick up small objects and crumbs between the thumb and finger. Provided they are first shown how, children are able to build a tower of two cubes and grasp a large crayon and scribble with it.

By 18 months the child should be able to walk well, start and stop safely, push and pull large toys and cardboard boxes around the floor and carry a large bear or other soft toy whilst walking. The child is able to run but in an awkward manner and is able to stop in front of furniture. Whilst the child is able to sit down by leaning backwards into a small chair, it will usually climb forward into an adult-sized chair and then turn round in order to sit. Balance is now sufficiently controlled to enable the child to pick up toys from the

Small muscle control.
(a) Placing one cube
on top of another
(15 months).
(b) Arranging cubes
horizontally
(18 months).

floor without falling over. The child can walk upstairs with the aid of an adult and crawl downstairs backwards, although it may prefer bumping down on its bottom.

Fine motor movements include spontaneous scribbling with a chunky pencil or crayon (and children may prefer to use one particular hand to do this), building a tower of three cubes, turning the pages of a book two or three at a time, pointing at pictures, holding a cup in both hands and drinking without excess spillage, using a spoon to get food into their mouths, and taking off their shoes, socks and hats.

Between 12 and 18 months the anterior fontanelle (which is the soft spot at the front of the skull) closes.

Intellectual development

Children show an even greater curiosity and experimentation through trial and error with different objects by using different aspects of their sensorimotor development. For example, if the child is in the playpen, it may experiment with various movements or objects to bring a toy from its position outside through the bars. Thus the child is demonstrating increasing control over its environment. Greater exploration is possible as the child is now able to crawl upstairs and walk a few steps. Adult supervision is required to prevent possible dangers in this extended environment, but this should not be obstructive or hinder the child's curiosity. Valuables and ornaments should be kept out of reach as the child will explore everything it finds. A large wheeled toy is popular as it aids independence in walking, and picture books are appreciated as they offer visual stimulation.

The child will take pleasure in imitating adult expressions and actions. If shown how to scribble it will use a crayon and copy and by 18 months will spontaneously scribble. At 15 months the child is often able to indicate when it has soiled its nappy but is not yet neurologically mature enough to be toilet trained. Hand preference is becoming more marked and should not be discouraged or altered. Myths abound about the merits of being right-handed, as in the past it was seen as a disadvantage to be left-handed. This may have originated from the Latin term for right, which is *dexter*, and people who are dexterous or have manual dexterity are admired within society. In contrast, the Latin term for left is *sinister* and this has negative connotations within our society. However, research has shown that hand preference is associated with the side of the brain that is most dominant, therefore those who are right-handed have a left-brain dominance and those who are left-handed have a right-brain dominance. The research has not shown that there is any difference in the abilities of left-handed and right-handed people. In fact in racquet sports it is a distinct advantage to be left-handed!

Language development

By the age of 18 months children will continuously talk to themselves in their own tuneful babble. They can use about 20 simple words but understand many more. They make their demands known by shouting, pointing or using simple words. The adult is able to help the child's language development by singing; reciting simple nursery rhymes which the child likes and will attempt to join in with; naming various parts of the body (hair, nose, arm, foot) and encouraging the child's efforts to demonstrate its knowledge of where the part is. Simple picture books are enjoyed and the child is able to point out simple objects as the adult talks and tells a story about the objects.

Language is more than speech as it involves cognitive development. Piaget maintained that the development of certain logical concepts frequently precedes the understanding of words corresponding to those concepts. Words such as 'bigger', 'smaller', 'longer', 'further' are not understood until the child understands the logical properties themselves. Language and thinking have separate roots and develop independently. The evidence of thought before language in the pre-verbal child is unquestionable and this can also be seen in children with learning disabilities who are able to answer questions about the content of their reading by pointing out the written word answer, despite their inability to verbalize more than two or three words.

Emotional development

As children struggle towards independence they are still emotionally vulnerable and require constant reassurance. At this stage they may develop anxiety when they are put to bed at night and will want a favourite toy or comforter; it is also important to leave on a night-light if they develop a fear of the dark. They may become clingier and want to be at the primary carer's side all the time or they may worry about strange places and new faces.

Social development

This is the stage just before temper tantrums when the child is striving for independence but feels vulnerable. The child may have developed a number of social relationships based upon its early attachments. Children seem to form relationships with those people who are particularly responsive to their signals for attention and the child will initiate social exchanges with them. Research has shown that the amount of time that the adult spends with the child is not the important factor but it is the quality of the experience for the child during the period of adult contact that is most significant.

Signs of Developmental Delay at 18 Months

Landers (1995) states that a doctor or health visitor should be consulted if the child shows any of the following signs of developmental delay at 18 months of age:

Fails to develop a mature heel-toe walking pattern after several months of walking

Does not speak at least 15 different words by 18 months
Does not use two-word sentences by age two
Does not seem to know the function of common household objects by 15 months
Does not imitate actions or words by the end of this period
Does not follow simple instructions by age two
Cannot push a wheeled toy by age two

(Landers 1995)

18–24 Months

Physical development

Children's mobility in crawling, walking and running allows them independence as they move around the home. They will enjoy running ahead of their care-givers on the way to the park, where they will show off new abilities in scaling the climbing frame or balancing on small benches or slides. They will like to join in ball games with friends and siblings, although they will still not be physically coordinated enough to throw balls. There is increased eye–hand coordination and this is demonstrated in their increased ability in reaching, grasping and manipulating objects by bringing them together and relating them to one another.

At 2 years children have reached a stage whereby they can run safely, avoiding obstacles and stopping and starting easily. They are able to rise to their feet from a sitting position without using their hands. They like to express independence through climbing on to furniture to look through a window or by opening cupboard doors and handling whatever comes to hand. When they walk upstairs and down they hold on to the rail or wall and put two feet on each step before moving forward. A small ball can be thrown but they will walk into a large ball when trying to kick it. Mealtimes also offer scope for more independence as they are able to lift and drink from a cup, replace it on the table and spoon feed themselves without spilling the food. The development of small muscle control is seen in the way the child removes wrappers, builds a tower of six or seven cubes, turns pages singly, scribbles spontaneously in circles and makes dots, imitates a vertical line and sometimes a letter V, puts on hat and shoes and is able to turn door handles.

Intellectual development

Piaget would now describe the child as passing from the sensori-motor stage to the pre-operational stage and intuitive thinking. At 18 months a child is aware of the practical relationships such as where objects are, where they were previously and where they belong. The child is able to indicate its nose, eyes, hair and shoes, and points to pictures of familiar objects such as a clock, a car or a dog. This transition from the sensorimotor to the pre-operational stage is characterized by symbolic games when the child imitates its own past actions in very simple, concrete ways which show that it has mental images of these actions, e.g. pretending to go to sleep, curling up its body and shutting its eyes. Children's imagination develops as they learn to pretend to drink first from a cup, then another object unlike a cup. With a vocabulary of about 15 words and an understanding of many more they are able to show appreciation of speech by imitating certain words and trying to join in nursery rhymes. They can undress themselves and are able to use a word in order to vocalize their need to use the toilet.

They are able to put large square, round and triangular pegs into matching holes and can make shapes from clay. They are able to draw horizontal lines and make a 'train' by placing blocks horizontally. At age two they are able to use a chair as a means to an end, e.g. pushing it over to a shelf and standing on the chair to reach something on the shelf. Imitation is shown in children's play when they copy the carer's domestic activities and they extend this symbolic play to their toys, which they pretend to put in bed to sleep. Piaget calls imaginative play 'the purest form of egocentric and symbolic thought'. Whilst it is egocentric in that the child is wrapped in its own dramatization, symbolic play leads it away from egocentricity because it enables the child to feel what it is like to be something or someone else apart from itself, e.g. a dog or an aeroplane. Egocentricity is a characteristic of the second major stage of intellectual development which Piaget calls the 'pre-operational thought period'.

Language development

At 2 years children will have a vocabulary of about 50 words and can understand many more. They are able to put words together to make simple sentences, e.g. 'Daddy go car'. Their curiosity seems insatiable as they continually ask the names of objects; the adult should answer questions in a meaningful way that can be understood by the child. Nursery rhymes, finger play, songs and pictures all help to stimulate the child's language.

Language development is dependent upon the child having a good learning environment and the interest of adults who will extend the child's language. Almost every part of the daily routine provides opportunities for extending children's vocabulary. The way adults speak to children and answer their questions will also have an effect upon children's linguistic development. By about 30–36 months, children will have a vocabulary of over 200 words. They will have struggled with the use of pronouns, recognizing themselves as 'I' (being the most important), then 'he', 'she', 'it', 'you', 'we', 'they' and 'us'. Familiar objects may be identified in pictures and their function given, e.g. ball – throw, bounce. They will also repeat words that they may have heard in conversation but they may not always understand the meaning of the words or where they should be used.

Emotional development

Children now experience and exhibit a variety of emotions (pleasure, satisfaction, joy, anger, frustration, distress etc.) as they struggle towards independence. They are still dependent upon adults for comfort and security, but the struggle between dependence and independence leads to temper tantrums. Temper tantrums are common between 18 and 36 months and need to be dealt with sensitively. Adults should not show anger during this phase as it is a normal developmental stage, but they can play a role in preventing tantrums. When dealing with a child in a tantrum the adult should adopt a friendly tone of voice, request the child to do something rather than command it, and say 'please' and 'thank you' to the child. Adults should not overreact when the child says 'No', and should not offer the child choices when none exist. Wherever possible the child should be offered alternative distracting activities and if necessary be taken out of the room away from other children and adults. Adults should choose battles carefully and should avoid situations that could lead to a tantrum. Good behaviour should always be positively rewarded. After the tantrum is over the child should be hugged to make it feel secure and to let it know that the normal relationship has returned unchanged.

Children will show pleasure in possessions which they label as 'mine'. They gain pleasure from achievements such as looking at pictures and pointing to and naming objects they recognize such as dog, bus or car. They like the comfort of sitting on the adult's lap.

Social development

Children's social development depends upon their home and environmental influences, for example whether they have siblings, live in a house or high rise apartment, meet other children in the park or at the one-o-clock club, or have a large extended family with grandparents, cousins etc. nearby. At this stage everything revolves around the child's world and it cannot understand the concept of sharing with other children. The child is content to play alongside other children but not with them (parallel play).

Toilet training

Toilet training must be a gradual process and should never become a 'battleground' between adult and child. Habit formation via routine in early infancy should have laid a foundation for the regularity of meals, nappy changing, bath times and sleep times. At 15 months some children will indicate when they are wet and at 18 months they may be able to indicate beforehand. Before toilet training children's physical development should be at a stage whereby they are able to sit comfortably on a potty and climb onto a chair. Negative reactions by carers to the child's lack of control can have an adverse effect on the child's learning abilities by causing feelings of guilt or making the child try too hard to please. It is helpful if the child is allowed to accompany a parent to the toilet in order to realize how natural it is. Bowel control is often achieved before bladder control, as there are fewer bowel actions for the child to cope with. Some children may be dry at night by $2\frac{1}{2}$–3 years; however, boys often take longer to achieve this than girls. Most children can keep dry during the day (with adult vigilance) by the age of $2\frac{1}{2}$–3 years.

When an accident occurs it is best to mop it up without comment; the child should not be scolded. Instead children should be praised when they warn you before the incident occurs, or even bring the potty to you. Patience and understanding are the prerequisites for the management of the 18-month-old child who is proceeding from the dependence of babyhood to the more independent toddler stage.

$2\frac{1}{2}$–3 Years

Physical development

At $2\frac{1}{2}$ years of age children can run well and climb simple apparatus. They jump with their feet together, are able to stand on tiptoe and can kick a large ball. They can walk upstairs on their own but need to hold a rail when walking downstairs and still do this by putting two feet on each step. They are able to push and pull large wheeled toys but they are unable to steer them around obstacles. They have now developed fine muscle dexterity and can pick up pins and thread, build a tower of seven cubes and arrange blocks to form a train. They are able to hold a pencil or crayon and imitate drawing a horizontal line, letters T and V and a circle, and paint strokes, dots and circular shapes using an easel. At the table they are able to use a spoon skilfully and may also be able to use a fork. They can pull their pants down to go to the toilet but find it difficult to pull them up again. In their sand and water play they enjoy filling jugs or other containers and tipping the contents out again.

By 3 years children can walk upstairs independently with alternating movements of the feet, although they will still come downstairs two feet to a step and are able to jump from the bottom step. They are able to climb apparatus at the nursery or swing park, can

*Building a tower of
seven pieces.*

push and pull large toys around corners and obstacles and can ride a tricycle and steer it around wide corners. They can stand on one foot and sit cross-legged. They are able to build small blocks into a tower of nine or make deliberate patterns with them. They can scribble freely, imitate circles, a cross, letters VHT, draw a man (usually a head and face with projections for arms and legs), can cut with scissors and can confidently paint pictures using a large brush. They are able to eat with a fork and spoon, and can carry their cup without spillage. They can wash their hands but need help with drying them. They are able to pull their pants up and down but need help putting on coats and fastening zips and buttons. They like to play with clay and dough, usually pounding and banging rather than making shapes.

*Intellectual
development*

The child's increasing body coordination is important for the development of intelligence at this stage as the sensorimotor schemes concerned with body control form the base for intellectual development. For example, the ability to grasp one cube and place it on top of another leads to the development of concepts such as 'under', 'over', 'on top' and the way in which the movement of the lower object causes movement of the upper object which is resting upon it.

Those who believe in Piagetian-based child development theory will argue that children must be encouraged to explore and discover properties of play materials. Therefore activities such as threading beads, music and movement etc. develop the child's understanding of space and time as well as helping the development of their fine motor movements. Pre-reading and pre-number activities, such as selection of clothes for dressing dolls and being able to put them on the doll in the right sequence, and setting the table with one plate and one mug for each child, are more important to children at this age than teaching formal reading skills.

At $2\frac{1}{2}$ years of age children engage in domestic play such as putting toys to bed and washing clothes. They are very jealous of adult attention and whilst they may show interest in other children they do not have the notion of sharing playthings. Developing curiosity is seen in the frequency of questions beginning 'What?' and 'Where?'. Children have no concept of time and everything happens in the present. However, they are beginning to see themselves as people and will ask 'Who?'. Children's motor ability enables them to build a tower of nine cubes, and after being shown a demonstration they are able to build a 'train' with a chimney and a bridge (two blocks placed side by side with one placed in the middle on top of both). They are able to discriminate between colours and can mix the primary colours (yellow, red and blue) to make new colours. They are able to match a circle, square and triangle on a form board.

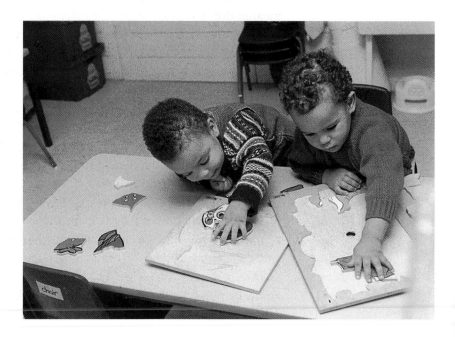

They are able to carry out requests to do small tasks and get a sense of satisfaction when they have completed these. They begin to join in activities with other children but still prefer solitary and 'parallel' play. Children gradually come to show an appreciation of past and present and will describe experiences of 'last night' and 'yesterday' although they do not at this stage understand the time concepts involved. They like to pretend to tell the time by asking 'What time is it?', 'When is lunchtime?'.

At this stage children are still marginally egocentric but as they progress further into the pre-operational phase new intellectual skills and knowledge enable them to predict other people's thoughts and feelings. However, children believe what they see, hear or experience at a given moment and are not able to apply what they have learned in previous situations to the present.

During the first half of what Piaget calls the preconceptual thought stage children are organizing their experiences into concepts such as time, space and number causality. In the second or intuitive phase they may be able to think in terms of grouping like objects together, such as 'apple, banana and orange are all fruit' but orange could also be put into the class of colour. The child will often use one word to describe a group of associated objects, for example calling all four legged animals dogs. Some children may refer to all men as 'daddy'.

For concepts of quantity children use words such as 'more', 'less', 'all', 'some' or 'none', as at this stage they are unable to count in a meaningful way. Concepts of number are linked with the Piagetian stage of concrete operations and children who seem able to count from one to 10 are probably just enjoying the rhythmic jingle without having a concept of 'oneness' or 'threeness' etc.

Language development

By the age of 3 years children are able to construct long sentences and can talk about situations in the past and in the future. They have a good command of vocabulary and this gives them confidence. Some children may have infantile substitutions for certain letters (usually p, t, th, f, s, r, l, w, y) and may say, 'I will wun' or 'I will go for a wide' or 'Give me dat' or 'Put it dere'. Children should not be corrected at this age as it will inhibit their free flow of conversation. Children's language will now develop in relation to their total behaviour patterns and the complexity or difficulty of the situations in which they find themselves and which they can deal with verbally. Starting at playgroup or nursery school will enhance their language development as they will learn new words alongside the new concepts.

Emotional development

This period is often described as 'the terrible twos' and/or the 'trusting threes'. At $2\frac{1}{2}$ years children are still swinging emotionally between positive and negative reactions. Sometimes they are rebellious, uncooperative and naughty and at other times they are dependent and clinging. Six months later they can be remarkably different, reacting in a cooperative, friendly and loving manner to adults and appearing to model themselves on adult behaviour. The $2\frac{1}{2}$-year-old can be aggressive and may quarrel noisily with another child if they are both trying to use the same toy. At this age children do not always distinguish clearly between people and things, both of which they consider to be their possessions. They are interested in other children but may regard them like curiosities by poking, pushing, hugging and even licking them (tasting them)!

At around 2 years children's imagination begins to develop. They may have dreams and nightmares and are unable to distinguish between fantasy and reality. When a child is 3 years their parents may have decided to have another child (a 3–4-year gap between children being the most popular in the UK). This may lead to the child experiencing sibling jealousy and rivalry. Jealousy arises when the child is frustrated by having to share the love of the parents and care-givers, whereas rivalry is the angry feeling which results when the child is frustrated in its desire to win. A new baby will make the youngest child jealous as it has been displaced from its position in the family and the feeling of rivalry may be felt towards an older sibling who is stronger and more able to cope, or the new arrival. Such feelings are quite natural and can be made less painful for the child if parents and care-givers are sensitive to the child's feelings. At any age a child should always be prepared in advance for the arrival of a new baby by parents and care-givers talking to the child, telling it stories, showing it pictures, pointing out other small babies and explaining to the child how dependent they are. Emphasis must be placed on the individuality of each child in the family and parents and care-givers should avoid competition or comparisons between children. It is also important to provide children with the right play experiences so they can work out their feelings through play.

Social development

Between $2\frac{1}{2}$ and 3 years is the time when most children will benefit socially by going to playgroup or nursery school. At this age they will usually attend for a morning or afternoon session. The mother or primary care-giver should always stay with the child when it first joins the group, as this will avoid the trauma of the first separation.

Slowly the child will come to trust the staff in the nursery or play-group, become interested in the toys and activities and will forget the presence of the mother or care-giver. It is at this point that the mother or care-giver can leave the child. It is important that the mother or care-giver is not late to collect the child at the end of the session; any lateness at this point will result in the child becoming distressed and feeling lost and abandoned.

3–4 Years

Physical development

Large muscle control is seen in children's ability to walk upstairs with alternating feet, march, run 10 steps with coordinated alternating arm movements, pedal a tricycle, somersault forward, kick a large ball when it is rolled to them, climb up and slide down a 1–2 m (4–6 feet) slide, jump from a height of 20 cm (8 inches), catch a ball with two hands and walk on tiptoe. The ability to use scissors has developed so they are now able to cut along a 20 cm (8 inch) straight line within 1 cm ($\frac{1}{4}$ inch) of the line. They are able to trace templates and put together a three-piece formboard or puzzle. Children this age have also developed further skills towards independence as they are able to use a knife, fork and spoon, brush their teeth, put on mittens, button and unbutton large buttons, put their coats on a hanger, and dress and undress themselves with some help with fasteners. All of the above indicate increasing development of the fine muscle movements and small muscle control.

Intellectual development

Children now have a large vocabulary of about 900 words and an understanding of many more. They will talk freely to themselves and others. Favourite words are 'Who?', 'What?', 'Where?' as they eagerly seek information about new aspects of their world such as the playgroup or nursery. Children's senses will add to their knowledge of the environment as they observe the actions of other children at play, and sometimes they will join in; they take part in music sessions and generally extend their play repertoire. Their liking for imaginative play is seen in their keenness to dress up and role play in the home corner. Their world of fantasy can be enhanced by stories, picture books, puppets, finger plays and songs. These children are now approaching Piaget's intuitive phase and beginning to form concepts as they play with sand, clay and water.

Time is first experienced in infancy as a series of events linked to the body rhythms and the patterns imposed by the environmental functions such as eating and sleeping. Later, actions which deal with a succession of objects, such as filling a cup with cubes at 18 months of age, or pushing and pulling a wheeled toy which starts and stops, all form the basis of time perception. Apart from the amount of time involved in these activities, the repetition of stimuli such as in music, dance or even rhythmically patting a baby in arms provides another kind of experience necessary for time concepts. An understanding of duration or an appreciation of the intervals in between events is also required for the development of a mature concept of time. Piaget states that the young child sees duration in terms of content rather than speed, which is the same idea we all share when it appears that pleasant events pass very quickly whilst painful or unhappy events seem to go on forever. At $3\frac{1}{2}$ years the child can use past and future tenses correctly and is able to use complex expressions of duration such as 'for a long time', 'for a whole week'. Children can tell their carers that they go to playgroup 'on Fridays' and that they played 'only for a short time' in the sand pit, but they may still confuse yesterday and today: 'I'm going for a walk yester-

SCENARIO 6.1

Jason is a child care student in a nursery school. Jason's tutor is paying a visit to the placement and asks Jason to describe the developmental value of outdoor play activities for 3–4-year-olds. Write an account of the answer that you would expect Jason to give to his tutor.

day'. Tomorrow and future events are well understood by 4-year-old children and they can recount recent events and experiences, although accounts are often a mixture of fact and fantasy.

It is important to note that children under 4 years of age cannot 'look forward' to events or even appreciate 'later this afternoon'. Adults often try to comfort 3-year-old children on their first day in nursery school with expressions like, 'Don't worry I will come back soon' or 'Don't worry I will be back at 3 o'clock', when children have no concept of 'soon', 'later' or '3 o'clock'. Children normally respond to these well-meant efforts by crying even louder as they see their carers disappear through the door in what to them is finality.

The child's concept of space is also derived from bodily experiences. In the sensorimotor stage children look, touch, grasp, feel, mouth and move arms and legs, fingers and toes and trunk in order to gain concepts of their body and other objects. In the pre-operational stage their concept of space is egocentric, i.e. related to their body movements and perceptions. The distance between the child and an object will influence the child's judgment of the object's size and the child's own size. The child tends to judge a close object as larger than it actually is and distant objects as smaller. Playing with blocks, trucks, tricycles and mobile toys helps children to perceive short distances accurately, but they cannot judge long distances unrelated to their own body size. Concepts of relative size enable children between the ages of 3 and 4 years to select the biggest and the smallest of a small selection of items.

Children's use of spatial terms is also linked with vertical orientation: for example when they are shown toy models of a dog and a horse they have no doubts that the horse is the biggest; however, if the dog is placed on a box making it higher than the horse they will say that the dog is the biggest, provided that they have seen the dog being moved. However, if at the start they are shown the animals with the horse on the ground and the dog on the box they will get the right answer by saying that the horse is the biggest. It would appear that moving the dog upwards whilst the child watches makes the child think 'vertically' and therefore 'big' means tall or high. Another explanation of this experiment is that the child does not understand the different concepts which are expressed by the words 'big' and 'high' or 'big' and 'tall' and therefore uses the wrong descriptor.

The concept of causality refers to the child's ability to explain events of the outside world. At the egocentric stage children explain everything in personal terms as they perceive them. Sometimes children will involve people close to them or, if they have been told about God, they will quote God as the cause of a number of events, so a 4-year-old child trying to explain 'night' says that 'God has put the lights out'. Of course this type of thinking stems from the explanations that adults have given to the child in answer to those 'Where?', 'How?' and 'Why?' questions. A more accurate answer about the reason for night from a child that has had its questions answered in an honest fashion may be 'The sun has gone to bed'.

Language development

By 4 years of age the child has a vocabulary of some 1500–2000 words, talks in sentences and continually asks questions. Language development during this period is rapid and the child talks, plays with words, comments, makes simple responses into long narratives, criticizes, balances comparisons etc. All situations are likely to be verbalized, even block play and drawing. The child's language is now moving beyond egocentrism and the immediate situation. The child is able to blend sounds together, an ability which is important for learning to read, and uses complete sentences, e.g. 'The tree is outside', 'The grass is wet'. The adult can learn a great deal by listening to the child's conversations with other children. If children are unable to communicate successfully with their peers then their self-confidence is likely to suffer.

Emotional development

At 3 years of age children emerge from their identity conflicts as trusting, generally friendly people who will now join in play with other children, show affection for younger siblings and be willing to share some of their toys. They like to help around the house and garden and reveal their feelings through imaginative play. As their self-confidence increases at 4 years, they may show reluctance to follow the wishes of an adult and give cheeky answers when reproved. Although they prefer to play with other children they are also capable of being aggressive towards them. They do learn to share and know that they cannot be first all the time and have to take turns with other children and share the attention of the adult. They are able to show compassion for other children by comforting a crying baby or a newcomer to the nursery. This compassion develops further as they get older. By 4 years children will not only be confident but also may be the seniors in the playgroup, and in this position may show a friendly, kindly interest in the younger children and enjoy being praised by adults for being 'sensible'. Children will model their behaviour on the adults around them; therefore if the adults present a confusing, inconsistent environment children will find it difficult to trust them. Even through they may be the 'seniors' children will still turn to adults for comfort when they are tired, hurt, afraid or ill.

Social development

The age of 3 years has traditionally been regarded as the ideal age for children to enter a playgroup or nursery school, as by this time they are ready to extend their social relationships. However, as mentioned earlier, some children may reach this stage at $2\frac{1}{2}$ years and others at 5 years.

At the 4-year-old stage, children tend to play in groups, but the focus of interest is the activity rather than the other children. These are not permanent groups; children will play together in a particular project, e.g. constructing a spaceship, then they will drift to another group for another activity. Four-year-olds like to tell long stories, often about everyday events, most of which are pure imagination. Some adults become annoyed when, having believed a story as the truth and maybe having taken action as a result of the events they have heard about, they have found out later from the child that it was pure fantasy. On the other hand some parents and carers will worry about children telling lies when they are indulging in their fantasy stories. A lively imagination is of great benefit to children as it enables them to solve problems of loneliness, jealousy and other matters that may be bothering them. Children will often invent an imaginary friend or companion; this may be in the form of a pet, adult or another child. Parents' carers and siblings are expected to accept the newcomer to the family and it will be the newcomer who will be blamed for naughty deeds and often used to draw attention to the child who may be feeling neglected. Alternatively the imaginary playmate may express the child's wishes to be grown up and powerful or naughty and babyish. Most parents and carers allow the child to outgrow the imaginary playmate, but if the playmate becomes too obstructive it may be necessary to set limits upon what it is allowed to do.

The socialization process by which children accept the customs, manners and traditions of the family, culture and peer group, enabling them to be accepted as members of society, involves two aspects that are sometimes seen as controversial: gender stereotyping and the idea that boys and girls are expected to behave differently. A lot has been written about both these areas and specific references can be found at the end of this chapter. Both parents and carers should give the same opportunities for play to boys and girls. Girls need the skills of learning to ride a bicycle and climbing as much as boys need the skills of cooking and learning to push a

SCENARIO 6.2

Maria is a nursery nurse in a nursery school. Eamon aged $4\frac{1}{4}$ years has thrown the Lego all over the floor and is refusing to pick it up. Eamon says that he did not do it but Curly did it. There is no child in the nursery called Curly. Write an explanation of what you think is happening here and how Maria should deal with Eamon.

pram. Children choose toys from interest, not because they are boys' toys or girls' toys. It is the influence of adults around them that will lead children to view certain toys as unacceptable. Small boys enjoy playing with dolls, but it is the negative reactions of their parents or carers which will lead them to believe that they should not play with dolls.

4–5 Years

Physical development

At this stage children develop and extend their existing skills. They are able to stand on one foot without aid for 4–8 seconds, are able to walk a balance beam, hop on one foot five successive times, jump backwards six times and jump forward 10 times without falling. Large muscle control is demonstrated when the child is able to run, change direction, jump over a string 5 cm (2 inches) from the floor, bounce and catch a large ball, walk downstairs with alternating feet and pedal a tricycle, which they can steer around corners. Manual dexterity is seen in their ability to make clay shapes which are put together in two or three parts, cut along a curved line, cut out a 5 cm (2 inch) circle, cut out and paste simple shapes and draw simple recognizable pictures such as a house, man or tree. Children can wash and dry their hands and faces, dress and undress alone, count the fingers on one hand using the index finger of the other hand, use correct utensils for eating food, carry out toilet activities unaided, put on and sometimes do up shoes (although for many children tying laces will be a skill at which they only become adept much later) and help set the table for meals.

Intellectual development

Between the ages of 4 and 5 years, after demonstration, children can build a tower of 10 blocks and any number of three-block bridges when requested. Building vertically is easier at this stage than making horizontal rows. It has been suggested that this may be due to the vertical space orientation of the body which remains constant in an up-and-down sense, whereas the environment of left and right sides changes constantly.

Dressing up activities provide opportunities for developing manual dexterity (4–5 years).

At age 5 years, children transfer from the nursery school or class into the infant school. This moving on should be a natural sequence and should not cause the child distress. The child should have previously visited the school and met with the head and class teacher. If children have not attended nursery school or playgroup then they are likely to find the transition to school a difficult and distressful event. As approximately 80% of all 4-year-olds are attending school either full time or on a sessional basis, it would be very rare to find a 5-year-old child who had no pre-school or school experiences. More details regarding the effects of school on children's intellectual development can be found in Chapter 7. They are able to join in group activities and like games which have rules (although they may choose to disregard these if they are not winning!). At this age children often

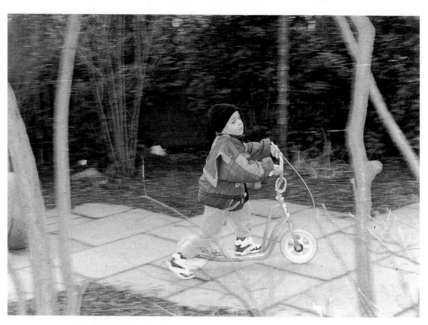

become bored with nursery activities and will need to be stretched intellectually to overcome this.

Language development

Children may have a vocabulary of around 3000 words, and ask many questions. They like to demonstrate their oral abilities and often test adults' reactions to 'bad language'. Parents and carers usually react with horror when a child uses a swear word and always insist that they did not hear it at home or nursery. Children are able to pick up swear words from radio, TV, listening to adults in shops and to other children. Parents and carers should not punish children for swearing; in the first instance they should ignore the child, but if it persists the child does need to be told that it is unacceptable language for the nursery or home. Children are able to classify in a more sophisticated manner, knowing the makes of cars, or names of flowers and trees, depending on where their special interest lies. Many children are interested in dinosaurs and it is interesting how they remember and correctly pronounce the very complicated names of the different types of dinosaurs.

Emotional development

At this age children are kind and protective towards younger children and pets. They enjoy stories that have strong and powerful people and they also like stories which have monsters and ghosts and may be scary but thrilling for them. They develop friendships with other children and want to be part of a group. They are beginning to understand that not all adults react in the same way and that adults have feelings too.

Social development

Between 4 and 5 years of age children may change from stable, friendly nursery 'seniors' into noisy, rude, boastful extroverts. This is often a defensive reaction to the major changes that they are undergoing as they enter school and find that the children there are so much bigger than they are. Peer groups now become very important and children are often motivated in their behaviour by peer group pressure and the need to have the approval of the peer group. Group games often become competitive, and the adult may need to act as the referee. They begin to understand cultural differences and that not all families are the same.

SCENARIO 6.3

Naghina is a student child care worker in a nursery school. The teacher has asked her to devise a project for a group of $4\frac{1}{4}$–5-year-olds. What developmental stages should Naghina take into account when devising the project?

5–6 Years

Physical development

When they reach primary school stage not all children have reached the same stage of development. There can be a wide variety of development stages in children of this age group depending upon their previous experience, environment and ability. Some children may appear to be ahead of others by being able to read, but it may also be found that these children may not be ahead in everything; for example they may be behind in manual skills and need help with dressing. For children in this position it can be very distressing to find that there are things they are unable to do; careful and sensitive handling is necessary as they will need a lot of encouragement. Most children have motor skills and control of their large muscles which enable them to: walk a balance board forwards, backwards and sideways; skip; swing on a swing initiating and sustaining motion; climb stepladders or steps to a slide; dribble a ball; kick a football; ride a bicycle; slide on a sledge; jump a rope; steer a wagon propelling it with one foot; walk or play in waist-high water in the swimming pool; jump up and pivot on one foot; jump from a height of 30 cm (12 inches) and land on the balls of their feet; stand on one foot without support and eyes closed; and hang from a horizontal bar bearing their weight on their arms.

Small muscle control enables most children to: spread their fingers; touch their thumb to each finger; copy small letters; print large capital letters anywhere on the paper; hit a nail with a hammer; colour in an outline staying within the lines for 95% of the picture; cut pictures from magazines or catalogue without being more than $\frac{1}{4}$ inch from the edge; use a pencil sharpener; copy complex drawings; tear simple shapes from paper; fold a paper square twice on the diagonal in imitation; catch a soft ball or bean bag with one hand; hit a ball with a bat or stick; print their name on lined paper; open a carton of milk; buckle their own car seat belt; and serve themselves and others with breakfast cereal.

Intellectual development

Starting school should promote the intellectual needs of 5-year-olds. At school they will learn to adapt skills which they practised at home or nursery such as eating, drinking, dressing, undressing, going to the toilet and washing their hands. Intellectual growth progresses with the maturation of the central nervous system. The 5–6-year-old age group marks a period of rapid physical and intellectual growth. The maturation process needs to be reached before a child can reach a developmental stage, and factors such as diet, poverty, wealth and environment may all have an effect upon the rate of maturation. Education is a stimulus for the growth of intelligence; however other factors also play a role, such as genetics, the experiences of the child etc. It is necessary for child care workers to recognize the differences in children's ability and accept that there is no educational process which can bring all children up to the same level. The effective child care worker, parent or teacher appreciates the differing ages, stages, interests and needs of all children in order that they can benefit as much as possible from their education.

As egocentrism decreases so children begin to see causes as impersonal and their understanding progresses from the concrete to a more abstract thought. This is the stage which Piaget referred to as the intuitive phase. At this stage children will explain events by a description or offer a number of different causes for an event, as they may have difficulty in understanding the concept of impersonal cause. Piaget described the tendency of children to attribute living qualities to inanimate objects as 'animistic thinking'. Adults often encourage children in this and television also encourages animistic thinking as children see stories of animated toys, trains and animals.

Piaget wrote about the child's stages of development in relation to the principles of conservation. Adults accept that the amount of a substance remains unchanged even when its shape is changed or when it is divided into parts. Children from 4–7 years do not have this concept. The child's conservation of mass can be demonstrated by giving a child some clay and asking him to make a ball the same size as an existing ball that he can see as a model. When the child is asked whether the two balls are of the same size he will reply 'yes'. One ball is then rolled into a long sausage shape and the child will now state that the sausage shape contains more clay than the ball because it is longer (therefore 'bigger' or 'more').

Language development

Children now have a large vocabulary that serves to unify the different aspects of their behaviour. They are able to count up to 10, know the names of the more familiar colours, and can give their name, age, birthday and home address when asked. They are also developing other skills relating to language such as listening, speaking, reading and writing. The child will learn and use new words learned at school and will also gain new words from books, poetry, stories and television.

Emotional development

Starting school may prove exciting and/or scary for children depending on their previous experiences away from home. Although the school may use informal learning methods there will be a lot of formal learning taking place alongside the informal. Children take a while to settle down, but once they have developed a trust and formed secure relationships with the teacher and the other staff they will regain their self-confidence. For many children the teacher becomes an important part of their lives, and many parents and carers will hear the teacher's thoughts on every subject from wellingtons to gerbils as quoted by the child.

Social development

Children who have had experience at nursery or playgroup will be used to making new friends and being away from their parents for part of the day. However, in spite of all the right pre-school experiences some children do not adapt to school. School can offer the excitement of new equipment and activities, but the child will get less attention from adults compared with the nursery. Teachers have considerable responsibilities to develop children's skills and teach them new knowledge and skills; carrying this out efficiently leaves very little time to spend on a one-to-one basis with individual children. Some children may miss this individual attention and this may lead them to behave in a way which attracts the attention of the teacher.

As the term proceeds so children will make friends and will introduce these friends to their parents or carers; they may be invited to

SCENARIO 6.4

Melanie has been learning in college about Piaget's theories relating to the child's development of the concept of conservation of mass. Devise an experiment that Melanie can use in her placement to illustrate Piaget's theory.

other friends' homes for tea or birthday parties. At this stage children are aware of the differences in adults and home life and are beginning to understand that they have to behave in a manner which is acceptable to a large number of adults.

6–7 Years

Physical development

At 6 years of age the average child is 1.07 m tall and weighs 18.14 kg. This is a period of rapid growth and 'filling out'; a similar process happens in adolescence. The development of motor skills during this stage depends less upon informal, spontaneous learning and more upon the learning of rules for formalized activities. There is now a change in the classroom setting and children have to sit longer and concentrate more on what they are learning. The child's muscle co-ordination and balance continue to improve as physical exercise is enjoyed for its own sake rather than as a competition with peers. Team games, e.g. football, rounders, skipping and hopscotch, are popular and both boys and girls should be encouraged to play all of these.

Intellectual development

The concept of conservation of weight and volume is more difficult than that of mass and most children cannot grasp this until they are 6 years of age or older. Children around the ages of 6–7 years can usually accurately answer the questions related to conservation shown in Box 6.1.

They are now not only able to recognize different shapes but know the properties of these shapes.

Language development

At this age children are able to recall part of a story, speak in sentences with more than five words, use the future tense and tell longer stories. They will speak up for themselves at the doctor or dentist and will enjoy making decisions. They have new words relating to mathematical and scientific concepts and are able to discuss these with adults. They enjoy conversations with their friends and like adults have an enjoyment for 'gossip' such as who has which new toy and where other children have been on outings or which TV programme they may have watched.

Box 6.1 *Conservation tests*

1. *Conservation of substance*
a. The adult presents two identical clay balls. The child agrees that they are equal amounts of clay.
b. One of the balls is rolled out to form another shape. The child is asked whether they still contain equal amounts.

2. *Conservation of length*
a. Two sticks are aligned in front of the child. The child agrees they are equal.
b. One of the sticks is moved to the right. The child is asked whether they are still the same.

3. *Conservation of number*
a. Two rows of counters are placed in one-to-one correspondence. The child admits they are equal.
b. One of the rows is spread out or brought closer together. The child is asked whether each row still has the same number.

Emotional development

At 6 years of age children can appear less stable than they were at 5 years of age. They may be irritable and self-centred and aggressively refuse to share toys and books. At times they may rebel against rules and the limits on behaviour set by teachers or parents. Children love to tackle new skills like computer techniques but they may become frustrated if they find them difficult.

Social development

This is the stage of Erikson's 'industry' versus 'inferiority' which lasts from 6–9 years, when the child's circle of significant relationships revolves around the school and the neighbourhood. During this phase children discover not only that they are distinct people but that they are able to do things by themselves or with others. They will take every opportunity to learn to become 'someone' in their imagination, such as a pop star, doctor, fire fighter, astronaut or police officer. They become very keen on the world around them and on gaining approval from adults.

Signs of developmental delay at 6 years

Landers (1995), whilst pointing out that each child develops in an individual manner, suggests that if a 6-year-old displays any of the following signs of possible developmental delay then a doctor or health visitor should be consulted:

Exhibits extremely fearful or timid behaviour
Exhibits extremely aggressive behaviour
Is unable to separate from parents without major protest

Is easily distracted and unable to concentrate on any single activity for more than five minutes

Shows little interest in playing with other children

Refuses to respond to people in general or responds only superficially

Rarely uses fantasy or imitation in play

Seems unhappy or sad much of the time

Does not engage in a variety of activities

Avoids or seems aloof with other children and adults

Does not express a wide range of emotions

Has trouble eating, sleeping or using the toilet

Seems unusually passive

Cannot understand two-part commands

Cannot correctly give her first and last names

Does not use plurals or past verb tense properly when speaking

Does not talk about her daily activities and experiences

Cannot build a tower of six to eight blocks

Seems uncomfortable holding a pencil

(Landers 1995)

7–8 Years

Physical development

Physical growth continues but not as rapidly as in the earlier stages. Physical skills increase through informal play and more formal games with rules and teamwork. This is a time when cooperation rather than competition should be encouraged in games. Very physical play such as that in adventure playgrounds should also be provided as this is an outlet for frustration and aggression.

Intellectual development

The stage from 7–11 years is Piaget's period of 'concrete operations' when the acquisition of concepts shows progression from the pre-operational thought period. Children are now able to classify (group objects or events with similar properties) and from this can understand the meaning of numbers and symbols. However, they will not be able to think of numbers hypothetically; they will still need concrete things to count. Concepts of colour are grasped more easily than concepts of form or shape. Learning to read and write demands attention to form and shape. Children have now reached a stage in development when they are able to sort by form or shape and then by colour; this also means that by the time they are 8 years old they are able to perceive form, colour and size in an abstract way. Concepts of direction are still difficult for children under 8 years. When they are asked where their home or school is they may be able to give the address, but actual directions may only be 'over there' or 'near the bus stop'. Children need to do a lot of work using real directional situations to help them to develop directional ability. Children only really understand the concept of right and left between the ages of 7 and 8 years.

Emotional development

Children now become increasingly confident as they become adept at new skills such as reading, writing, tying knots and bows, climbing trees, swinging or ropes and balancing on the equipment in adventure playgrounds. They like stories about the wonders and myths of magic, wizards, heroes and heroines and fables. They enjoy dramatic interpretation and may need restraining from too literal a translation of their particular idol's pursuits! This stage of development is a time of great joy and enthusiasm for life and the discovery of nature and the world around them. At this stage children begin to become aware of morality, i.e. knowing the difference between right and wrong.

Social development

Both girls and boys adopt heroes and can reel off the names of current pop stars, football stars, TV personalities etc. Children of this age like to write and receive letters; this may need some encouragement at first but they get great pleasure from receiving their own letters through the mail box. Children also know that letters are a good way of conveying thoughts and feelings to others and thus being able to share pleasures. Some children may appear to be natural leaders and this should be discouraged as it is important that leadership is shared. The school should offer a climate of cooperation rather than competition.

ASSIGNMENTS

1. Choose two well known child development theorists and give a brief résumé of their theories.

2. What might be the signs of developmental delay in a child aged 18 months?

3. Why are the expressions 'terrible twos' and 'trusting threes' used to describe children aged 2 years and 3 years?

4. Describe the language development of a 4-year-old.

5. What does Piaget's stage of 'concrete operations' mean?

6. Write an essay on why it is important for children to learn to be cooperative rather than competitive.

PRACTICAL ACTIVITIES

1. Undertake five observations of a 3-month-old baby. Compare your results with the information on development in this chapter and Chapter 5. From the comparison write an evaluation of the observations.

2. Observe two new children on their first day at nursery school or playgroup. Evaluate their reactions and comment on any differences you observed between the children.

3. Prepare an activity for a group of 4-year-olds and clearly state the aims of the activity in terms of their physical, intellectual, linguistic, emotional and social learning.

4. Set up the water trolley for a group of 3-year-olds and put new water play equipment out that they have never used before. Observe how the children play with this equipment and how they solve problems/find explanations as to how the equipment works.

5. Keep a diary over a two week period spent in your setting. Record all the 'How', 'Why' and 'What' questions that the children ask during that time. Evaluate your findings to see if there are particular groups of questions which are asked more frequently than others.

References

Bee H 1992 The developing child, 6th edn. Harper Collins, New York

Landers C 1995 Childhood trainers: guide to the development of the young child. In: Enhancing the skills of early trainers pack. Bernard van Leer Foundation/UNESCO, Holland

Leach P 1997 Your baby and child: the essential guide for every parent. Penguin, London

Martorano SC 1977 A developmental analysis of performance of Piaget's formal operations tasks. Developmental Psychology 13:666–672

Qualifications and Curriculum Authority and DFEE 1999 Early Learning Goals. QCA Publications

Further reading

- Browne N, France P 1986 Untying the apron strings: anti-sexist provision for the under fives. Open University Press, Milton Keynes

- Dunn J, Kendrick C 1982 Siblings: love, envy and understanding. Grant MacIntyre, London

- Faragher J, MacNaughton G 1990 Working with young children: guidelines for good practice. TAFE Publications, Victoria, Australia

- Fatchett A 1995 Childhood to adolescence: caring for health. Baillière Tindall, London

- Grabrucker M 1988 There's a good girl: gender stereotyping in the first three years of life: a diary. The Women's Press, London

- Gross RD 1992 Psychology: the science of mind and behaviour. Hodder & Stoughton, London

- Leach P 1989 Baby and child: from birth to age five. Penguin, London

- Lindon J 1993 Child development from birth to eight: a practical focus. National Children's Bureau, London

- Phillips A 1993 The trouble with boys: parenting the men of the future. Pandora, London

- Reid J 1995 More than meets the eye. New research into babies. Nursery World 23 November: 12

- Sheridan M (Revised and updated by Frost M, Sharma A) 1997 From birth to five years: children's developmental progress. Routledge, London

- Williams K, Gardner R 1994 Caring for children. Pitman Publishing, London

Chapter 7

Children's Play and Education

This chapter covers underpinning knowledge for parts of the following units for the National Vocational Qualifications (NVQs) in Early Years Care and Education: C8, C9, E1, M7. This chapter is also linked to the following CACHE Awards Units: Diploma Units 2,6; Certificate Units 2, 3.

INTRODUCTION

Friedrich Froebel (1782–1852) was probably one of the first people to recognize that children's play was more than just something that the child did in order to pass the time; it was actually a serious and deeply significant activity for young children. Susan Isaacs (1885–1948) wrote:

> If we were asked to mention one supreme psychological need of the young child, the answer would have to be 'play' – the opportunity for free play in all its various forms. Play is the child's means of living and of understanding life.

> (Isaacs 1954)

In 1987 John Brierley, through careful study of the development of children's brains, stated:

> All forms of play appear to be essential for the intellectual, imaginative and emotional development of the child and may well be necessary steps to a further stage of development.

> (Brierley 1987)

A further acknowledgement of the importance of play is reflected in the United Nations Convention on the Rights of the Child (1989), Article 31, which states:

> Every child is entitled to rest and play and to have the chance to join in a wide range of activities.

From the above quotes and the significant contributions made by their authors to the field of child development there can be no doubt of the effects of play upon the child's psychological, intellectual, linguistic, emotional and social development.

As play is a powerful medium for learning it is important that all child care workers understand the value to the child of different types of play and how to present play activities that are appropriate to a child's stage of development. Through play children learn skills, gain concepts and understanding and draw relationships between concepts. They are able to practise problem solving and decision making, and learn how to successfully interact with other children and adults. They are able to build up their vocabulary and learn to express their ideas in words. There are four essential provisions needed for a child to have good play and learning experiences:

- A range of rich experiences
- An environment with interesting material and equipment relevant to the age and stage of development of the child
- An atmosphere in which each child is allowed to proceed at its own pace
- Understanding adults who are able to facilitate meaningful play experiences for the child.

ROLE OF THE ADULT IN PLAY

The adult has an important role in providing an interesting, safe and suitable play environment for the child. There should be adequate space for the child to be able to manipulate equipment. Whilst the adult will structure some of the play activities there also need to be other materials that are easily accessible for the child to introduce into the activity. For example, the adult may have set up the water-play area with the appropriate equipment to enable the child to strain, float, sink, pour, turn waterwheels etc. However, the child may decide to introduce some bricks in order to build a dam or use the water to wash the dolls and this will only be possible if the child has easy access to the bricks and dolls. If children do not come up with their own ideas for extending the play activity then the adult may offer suggestions. In this instance the adult's role is that of a facilitator who is able to provide an activity, observe and listen to the way the children use the activity and if necessary offer some new ideas in order to make the activity more challenging for the children.

Adults do need to intervene in children's play when it becomes dangerous or too boisterous, and in this case the role of the adult is to set boundaries or limits upon the children's actions or behaviour. The adult has a role in listening carefully to the children's use of language whilst they are playing and offering new words and descriptions.

Athey (1990) maintains that if adults observe children they will notice that the child exhibits 'a pattern of repeatable behaviour into which experiences are assimilated' and she calls these 'schema'. Athey identifies seven types of schema:

- Dynamic circular
- Dynamic vertical
- Dynamic back and forth, side to side
- Going over and under
- Going round a boundary
- Enveloping and containing
- Going through a boundary.

The role of the adult is to recognize the schema and provide activities for the children that will enable them to pursue their particular schema. For example, if children are working on a schema of enveloping and containing they will need activities which will enable them to extend the schema such as empty boxes, digging in the garden, wrapping parcels, putting dolls to bed etc.

A great deal of nursery practice requires the adult to be 'non-directive' and the activities to be 'child directed'. This usually means that the adult's role is to provide a stimulating environment and interesting materials and equipment to which the child will respond if it wishes. This view overlooks the very important role that adults can play if they become involved in children's play. Materials should be made available in such a way that the children's curiosity leads them to explore, discover various properties of the play equipment, and ask questions about their findings. The adult helps the children clarify concepts and corrects misconceptions. Provision for individual differences in the child's learning style and rate are made as the adult helps the child towards problem solving in a way that corresponds to the child's developmental stage.

It is often difficult to determine the difference between a positive form of intervention and the adult interfering in the child's play. If comments are made too often, children become dependent upon the adult and stop playing when the adult moves to another group. If there is too much adult interference the children will lose interest and ownership in the play.

Adults' questions to children should be open ended (i.e. not allowing a 'yes' or 'no' or one syllable answer) in order to extend the children's language and thinking. Examples of open ended questions could be:

- 'What are you going to do with this?' (stating the problem)
- 'How will you manage to put all those bricks into the wheelbarrow?' (testing understanding)

- 'Why did you have two wheelbarrows yesterday?' (recall)
- 'What do you think will happen if you pile them all in the small wheelbarrow?' (prediction)
- 'Why did we need two wheelbarrows yesterday?' (recap process)
- 'Which way is easiest for workers to move all these bricks?' (imaginative).

Any comments made by the adults should extend the child's learning, encourage thinking and clarify concepts.

When adults answer children's questions they must be honest in their answers. When adults do not know the answer to a child's question then they should tell the child that they do not know and suggest setting up an experiment to find out, or go together to the library to look up the answer. This does mean that child care workers need to understand the concepts themselves, such as why different objects sink and float, why plants cannot grow without light, what happens to the hamster when it dies, and how aeroplanes fly. Due to the influence of media such as television many more children are very knowledgeable about a great number of things and this can lead to children asking very sophisticated questions for which they want answers.

Imaginative play offers a lot of scope for adult involvement if adults are invited by the children to join in the game. Children often invite adults into the home corner for tea or to buy goods at the classroom shop. Involvement in imaginative play enables the adult to extend the children's verbal skills and add an extra dimension to the imaginative process.

Repetition of routine activities will provide a sense of security for young children, but the timetable must be flexible to enable children to finish a project or go on outings or enjoy spontaneous play.

The adult has a role in the organization and supervision of children's play. Staff should work as a team and plan activities at least 1 week ahead. Many nursery schools and classes will have long term activities such as outings, concerts and sports days, which have to be slotted into the timetable throughout the year and may not fit with the learning theme for a particular term.

Activities are usually organized on a monthly or weekly basis and are planned to fit in with the learning theme. With the emphasis now being on the early years, curriculum activities are often accompanied by the learning outcomes or goals for the children. Some early years establishments with 4-year-olds are likely to be working towards the national desirable learning outcomes for children's

SCENARIO 7.1

You are a nursery nurse in a local nursery school working with a group of 4-year-olds. Part of your role is to work with the teacher in planning activities for the children. Activities are usually based upon a theme; the theme for this term is Winter. The teacher has asked you to draw up a list of activities for 1 week based upon this theme and to state the likely learning outcomes for the children.

learning on entering compulsory schooling, which are assessed when the child reaches infant school. (Further reference to these is made later in the chapter.)

Planned learning outcomes should be achievable by the majority of children. Special needs children in the nursery may need extra help in order to achieve specific outcomes. Examples of learning outcomes are as follows:

- Recognizing the motif on their own coat peg
- Counting to five and having an understanding of fiveness
- Identifying the colours blue, red and green.

Activities will be chosen that will give the children the knowledge and skills needed to achieve the outcomes. For example, in learning to count to five and understand fiveness they will learn rhymes, songs, stories that involve numbers and counting, activities using five bricks, playing in groups of five children, cooking five cakes, learning the names of five days of the week etc.

Careful observation of a child's activities enables the adult to approach the child at the right level and enables the child to utilize its experiences with various materials. The adult can encourage children to discuss their work, although adults must be careful not to make negative remarks about the work, as this will damage the children's self-confidence.

Adults also have a role to ensure that the play environment is safe, removing broken toys, leaking water trays etc.

DEVELOPMENT THROUGH PLAY

As already stated, play is the child's main medium for learning and as such has implications for all aspects of development. All activities that the child undertakes are learning situations, therefore adults should never say, 'We'll finish this first and then you can play' as this draws an unnatural divide which suggests that some activities are more important than others, e.g. reading books is learning whereas dressing up is play.

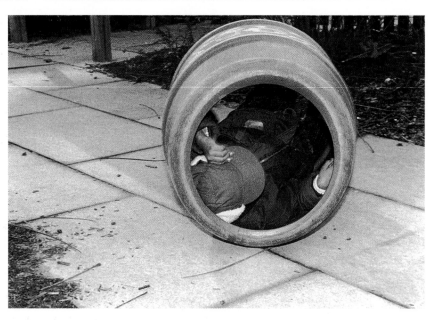

Physical Development

Children benefit from play as it helps them to acquire body control. Coordination develops through movement and exercise. Random movements become purposeful as the child grasps a moving object. Later children progress from crawling to walking and running, from standing on one foot to hopping; and eventually to more complicated games requiring physical skills with large and small muscle movements.

Intellectual Development

Children are able to develop new skills and abilities with words and objects, experiment with the properties of creative media and play equipment and solve problems in their own way. Exploratory play begins at the breast with the most primitive senses of touch and taste, then proceeds through random movements to voluntary control of the hands, arms and legs which enables the child to grasp, hold and examine small objects. Through these movements the baby comes to acquire control over its body and attempts to control the environment as it progresses from crawling to walking and running. Babies discover textures of food and other materials first by putting them in their mouths, later by feeling and close examination. Different shapes and sizes come to recognition as they try to grasp the coloured mobiles strung above their cots. Experimentation begins as they pull the cord that will set the chime bar into action and introduce another dimension, sound, into the activity.

Play with sound develops with the child's own babbling which is obviously a pleasurable activity apart from its later significance as a means of communication. Concepts of colour, form and size and properties of different play materials lead children to classify and categorize items to their own criteria. Eagerly they question in their enthusiasm to learn. A discovery such as the necessity to add water to sand before one can build with it is as important to the child as any discovery made by Archimedes. Emotional aspects are closely interwoven in children's pride at achievement, and the adult should express the appropriate appreciation of their efforts.

Emotional Development

Play provides an outlet for feelings and children can use playthings on which to vent their anger; smacking teddy, kicking the ball or pounding clay is preferable to the child punching other children or adults, or breaking plates and ornaments. As they develop they learn to use anger in a constructive way, hammering nails into wood or making clay models.

Play involves not only the negative feelings of fear, aggression, anxiety, hate, guilt and frustration, but also pleasure, happiness, exuberance, love and affection. Sometimes children have ambivalent feelings towards their parents; 'I don't love you anymore' or 'I hate you' are often said by children as they enter a power struggle which may revolve around a simple matter such as parents not allowing them a second slice of cake. Sometimes children will turn towards quiet peaceful activities such as jigsaw puzzles, stacking toys, Lego, water play or the book corner. This ability to use objects for their own needs will enable children to cope with difficulties in future life.

Language Development

Play is a very powerful tool for the development of children's language. Bee (1992) points out that a number of researchers have noted the relationships between the patterns of children's play and their language development. Through play children develop new concepts, and with each concept there is a set of associated descriptive words. Young children may often have a gap between the number of concepts which they have and the number of words at their disposal to describe these concepts. In other words, children often have an understanding of more concepts than they are able to describe. As children learn new words they incorporate these into their play and the play becomes more complex. Children often understand many more words than they are able to speak. Children may use language in their play in order to develop social relationships with other children and with adults. Through play children are able to practise their language ability, and particular types of play, for example doll play, home corner, cooperative play and imaginative play, offer opportunities for the child to try out new words and sentences. Adults have an important role in extending children's language through play activities and introducing new words. Through play children are able to learn the language of problem solving, with the adult answering questions and offering simple explanations for the 'how', 'why', 'what' questions. As they get older (4–5 years old) children will use language in play situations to ask complicated questions, to negotiate with other children, to explain what they are doing or what they intend to do next, to express their thoughts aloud, and to give instructions to others. Between the ages of 6 and 8 years they will use language to introduce rules into their games and ensure that all players keep to the rules.

Social Development

The process of socialization develops throughout the child's life. In the first years of life, children learn to socialize with the immediate members of their own family; when they go to playgroup or nursery they learn to socialize with other children and adults outside the family circle. Many children soon discover in this situation that what has been acceptable behaviour within their own family is not always acceptable outside of the family. Children will need to learn how to play cooperatively with their own peers as well as how to interact with adults such as teachers and playgroup and nursery workers. This will be their first introduction to the rules and expectations of a wider society. They must learn to share, take turns, communicate with children and adults and negotiate their way into games and activities, which is often more complex than just saying 'May I play too'. Having negotiated themselves into a game or activity, children then have to learn and apply the rules that appertain to the situation; those who do not manage to do this will be viewed as spoiling the game. They have to become aware of and understand the feelings of others, understanding when they may be hurting other children or being unkind to them. The adult has an important role to play in this as most children learn by observing and adopting the example offered by the adults around them.

VALUE OF DIFFERENT TYPES OF PLAY

Imaginative Play

This helps children gain pleasure, learn self-expression and explore and solve problems, and enables them to pass from the egocentric stage to objectivity. Pretence and symbolic play are early forms of representation, and fantasy play helps children cope with emotions and problems in childhood.

Fantasy play can start as early as 18 months, but well formed pretend play usually appears around 3 years of age. From the age of 7–8 years, fantasy play begins to diminish as the child's reasoning ability and experience leads it to distinguish between fantasy and reality. However, many adults still appreciate the opportunity to indulge in fantasy play, hence the large number of amateur dramatic societies which flourish around the country. In imaginative play children rehearse their interests, skills and obligations, and make experiments in social relationships without having to pay the penalty for mistakes.

Symbolic play enables children to relive their past experiences, and in older children the symbols are replaced by rules in social play. Role play refers to any activity in which the child assumes a distinct identity different from its own; this is a special category of pretend or make-believe play. In role play the child will announce, 'I am the doctor, Robin is the nurse and Lee is the sick person'. In pretend or make-believe play the child will say, 'I am driving my ambulance to the hospital' whilst sitting on a wooden truck.

Dressing-up clothes, cardboard boxes, blocks, household equipment etc. will be the only materials that children will need to indulge in imaginative play. A piece of highly coloured cloth can as easily be used as a sari as it can a bridesmaid dress. Hats and bags are useful items for encouraging make-believe or role play. Role-playing television and film heroes is a very common type of pretend play amongst 4–5-year-olds; they love to indulge in being a super-hero for a morning.

As well as aiding social and emotional development, imaginative play develops eye–hand coordination and small manipulative skills which are needed to put on and take off clothes, concepts of size and number and sequential order being developed through the play itself. When imaginative play is in groups, social development is aided as children play cooperatively and exchange ideas and take turns in being superheroes.

Constructive/ Manipulative Play

Constructive play enables the child to experience the satisfaction of producing an end product. For the younger child the activity is more important than the end product. Children begin to construct and manipulate materials by using dough, clay, sand, blocks, wood, scissors, paste, crayons etc. They may use their construction as part of their imaginative play. When children first use manipulative play they will not have an end product in mind, although if asked they are likely to make a last-minute decision as to what the construction represents. As they get older and use sophisticated construction toys such as Lego they may have a very definite end product in mind. Older children are capable of producing very complex constructions using blocks, Lego, junk materials etc. Whatever children produce in their constructive activities must be appreciated and acknowledged by the adult as it would have been made with a lot of thought and effort. Sometimes children will need encouragement to complete a construction and the adult may need to offer suggestions as to how best this can be done. Such a timely intervention may help the child to learn not to opt out when things get difficult. Children can become very absorbed in constructive play and spend long periods of concentration on the activity. Constructive play allows opportunities for solitary, parallel and cooperative play. It is important that the adult does not discourage them; there is nothing more frustrating for children than being asked to pull apart a construction because it is lunchtime. It is important to have a safe place to keep a half-completed construction so that the child can come back to it after lunch or the next day.

Block Play

The block area should be sited out of the way of traffic in the nursery so that the children can build without interference from others and their construction does not prevent other activities from taking place. The block storage cupboard should be low enough to enable the children to manipulate the blocks in and out of the cupboard and should have sufficient shelves to store blocks of similar shapes together. Large unit blocks allow children to discover equivalences and other mathematical relationships as well as giving children an understanding of space and area.

Block play encourages physical development and the children's gross motor skills as they bend, lift, stretch and crawl. As they handle each block so they are developing fine muscle control and eye–hand coordination. Control of the fingers and hand is seen in the palmar grasp for large blocks and the pincer grasp for the smallest blocks. Balancing on constructions such as 'bridges' promotes foot control, as does standing on tiptoe to reach high blocks.

From blocks, children discover concepts relating to size, shape, position, weight and height. Where the shape of the block is drawn on the shelf to correspond to the position of the block, children are able to relate a two-dimensional drawing with a three-dimensional object as well as learning to identify a block by a symbol. Activities in block play offer the child the opportunity to develop concepts which are the basis of maths, language, physics and social development. Learning that certain blocks stack more easily because they are of a similar shape, a child can stack in a progressive series of size, practise one-to-one correspondence by piling one block onto another, learn that blocks are the parts which go towards making the whole structure of a tower or bridge, and learn how to take away blocks to make a structure lower and how to solve problems. Block play increases children's vocabulary as they learn the meanings of words such as higher, lower, smaller, larger, skyscraper, factory, bridge, tower etc.

Blocks, as constructive play, enable children to produce something to their own specifications and this gives them an enormous sense of pride. They develop self-confidence as they learn to manipulate the blocks and get a feeling of satisfaction when they knock down something that they have created. Block play is an activity which allows children to play in groups, sharing ideas, respecting each other's opinions and contributions and problem solving together. It also offers the opportunity for children to play alone, and some days they will play in a group while other days they will play alone.

Creative Play

Creativity involves discovery, invention, experience, imagination, experimentation, problem solving and establishing new links between what already exists, e.g. a blanket, table and chair can become a cave for exploring. If creativity is to be fostered in the nursery, the attitudes of the staff must allow for children to deviate from the 'norm', as one original piece of work is far more valuable than 20 pieces of work based on an adult-made template. Apart from the obvious creative activities such as painting, collage, junk modelling (see Box 7.1), dough and clay, there are other activities which develop children's imagination and enable them to express their creativity, such as music and movement, dramatic play, dressing up etc. Adventure playgrounds provide scope for free expression and aid development of imagination and creativity with their tyre swings, tree trunks, rope and metal climbing frames, barrels etc.

In using creative materials such as dough, clay and wet sand, children learn about the properties of natural materials and how these can be manipulated in order to form an end product. They learn about the use of symbols (square for a house, circle for the sun) to represent real objects. The production of pictures and patterns develops the child's aesthetic appreciation. The adult can help develop the children's imagination by extending their experiences with outings, classroom displays, colourful picture books, providing interesting materials such as glittery paper, pieces of exotic material such as silk and satin, corrugated paper, gold and silver foil etc.

Adults should never comment on the artistic value of what the child has produced but must be non-judgmental, appreciating that for the child it is the process that is important and not the product. Every child's work should be put on display, and adults who are skilled at mounting and displaying children's work can make even the poorest effort look splendid.

Box 7.1 *Items to collect for the junk table*

Aluminium foil	Elastic	Ping pong balls
Beads	Fablon	Pipe cleaners
Birdseed	Feathers	Plastic and
Books	Felt	polystyrene trays
Bottle tops	Fir cones	Plastic bottles
Braid	Foam rubber	Polystyrene
Brushes	Foil dishes	Raffia
Buttons	Fringes	Ribbon
Candles	Glitter	Rice
Cardboard	Grasses (dried)	Sand
Cards (birthday,	Ice lolly sticks	Sawdust (can be
Christmas, holiday)	Insulating tape	coloured with
Cartons	Jewellery	food colouring or
Cellophane (off	Kitchen roll centres	powder paint)
sweets, etc.)	Lace	Seeds
Cereal packs (cut to	Leather	Sequins
give a good solid	Leaves	Sheep's wool
base)	Lino (scrap)	Shells
Chalk	Lolly sticks	Shoe boxes
Cheese boxes	Magazines (for	Silver paper
Christmas paper	cutting out)	Squeezy bottles
Coat hangers	Margarine	Straw
Cocktail sticks	containers	String
Coloured paper	Match boxes	Sweet papers
Corks	Material (scrap)	Tape
Corrugated paper	Meat trays	Threads
Cotton reels	Melon seeds	Tiles (ceiling)
Cotton wool	Milk bottle tops	Tissue boxes
Crayons	Net bags	Trimmings, e.g. lace,
Doilies	Netting	braid, ric-rac
Dried	Newspapers	Velcro
coffee granules	Nut shells	Wallpaper (rolls and
egg shells	Paper	old books)
melon seeds	Paper plates and	Wood
sand	cups	Wood shavings
tea leaves	Pebbles	Wool (used and new)
Egg cartons	Pine cones	Yoghurt cartons

In painting and creative activities, children develop fine muscle control through management of the brush, using different parts of the body to paint with (e.g. foot painting) and controlling the amount of paint that they will use. The children are able to make decisions as to where on the paper they will start, what the end product will be, or what character they will dress up as. They will experiment with paint, mixing colours together; they will try modelling with wet and dry sand and learn that you cannot model with dry clay. Children get great enjoyment from this experimentation process; it can be very satisfying for a child to find out what it is like to walk in high-heeled shoes or wear a wig. Children can express themselves through creative activities, particularly releasing strong feelings when slapping paint on paper, banging dough, hammering wood and nails. These activities allow children to work at their own pace, either alone or with others.

Stages of development in children's painting

Rhoda Kellogg (1955) carried out studies of children's drawing in Africa, Japan, Tonga, Austria and England, and found that all children react to paint in the same way. If given something to draw with and something to draw on they will discover by themselves and then use similar drawing symbols. Patterns of development are clearly seen in the universality of the symbols which they use and the order in which they use them. It does not matter at what age children have their first experience of drawing, they will go through the same development stages using the same symbols. Obviously for an older child with greater muscle control many of these stages will be passed through very quickly.

Almost all children begin drawing by scribbling and as Jameson (1973) points out, they may use any medium to do this, 'fingers in food, sticks in dust or sand, steam on the window, but they soon graduate to more positive media like crayons, chalk, pencil on

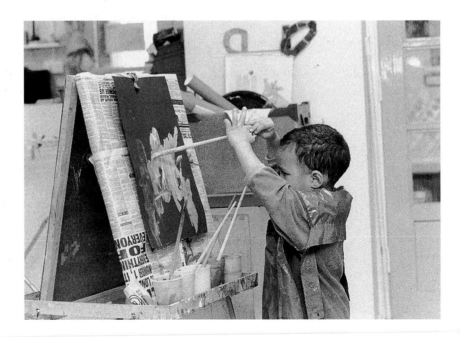

blackboard or wall paper in the sitting room or … large sketch books or pads.' They will continue to scribble until they move towards a shape, usually an oval. Children then develop the oval into a house, a cat, or a bird, anything they want to develop it into. From the oval the child develops what Jameson describes as the radial; this is where the child has added radii coming out from the oval. Children begin to use the oval as the head and the radii as arms and legs (not necessarily in the correct numbers). In order to develop the head the child will add dots in a circle for eyes, a mouth depicted by a line of scribble and a circle on each side of the oval to depict ears. The number of radii diminishes so there are two representing legs and sometimes there will also be two for arms. Children will use this figure for playing out fantasies and symboliz-ing their experiences.

The next stage of development is when children begin to experi-ment with paint. The first stage is when they make blobs of colour on the paper indicating that they have found the paint and are manipulating the paint and brush to connect with the paper. They find they can create different colours by mixing one on top of the other on the paper. They then discover that by using each individ-ual brush that is in each pot of paint or washing their brush before going to a new colour they can create more distinct colours which resemble colours in the environment. They learn to manipulate the brush from scribble movements, to dots, to patches. They will fill the whole paper with patches of colour. In order to do this, children need skill and coordination, and need to make choices. They will aesthetically superimpose one colour on top of another in order to create colourful patterns. They will become more controlled in their application of colour, sequencing colours and shapes.

The next stage is when they connect the use of paint and their drawings of the oval and radii to produce what Jameson describes as a colourful 'big head'. They use this to symbolize their experi-ences. The 'big head' then moves through the arms and legs stage and the children add a body by using a patch of colour. The body may then be given arms, the head will be given hair and by around 5 years of age children will be painting fingers at the ends of arms and toes or shoes at the ends of legs.

Once they have become confident in drawing the figure they will progress to painting the 'house'. This starts out as an empty square with patches of colour for the windows. They will slowly add new symbols to the house, e.g. squares for window glass, a chimney and a door, so that the painting of the house becomes more sophisticated and complex. They may even add the sun, rain, trees, or turn the house into a caravan by giving it wheels. They will also give complicated explanations of their paintings, often telling the adult the story attached to the symbols. By the age of 6–7 years their drawings have become quite detailed and sophisticated with large buildings, many people, cars, aeroplanes, cats, dogs, rainbows, snow etc. And there is evidence of a lot of activity happening in the pictures. Their paintings represent the things that they have seen around them or may be part of a project such as dinosaurs, zoo animals etc.

Books and Storytelling

Children's knowledge and creative thinking are encouraged and developed by books and stories. Children not only get a great deal of enjoyment from books but they also benefit emotionally, intellectually, socially, linguistically and culturally. Feely books can offer young children tactile experiences as can books made of different materials such as cardboard, cloth, plastic inflatable floatable books etc. For very young children, books should have large clear illustrations of familiar objects or animals in primary colours, with no or few written words. Pictures must be complete, cars must have four wheels and animals must have a head, body and four legs. At this age, books are to look at and the adult can talk to the child about the pictures in the book; it is not necessary to have a story line.

It is a pleasant emotional experience for children to be sat on an adult's lap looking at a book while the adult reads the story. They

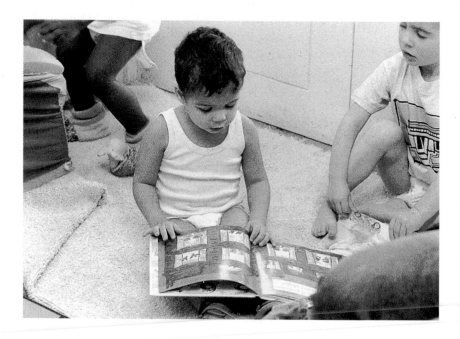

feel safe and secure and they like to ask for their favourite story to be read over and over again. In the school or nursery there should be a book corner which should appear warm and inviting with a carpet, low shelves so that the children can reach the books, and small comfortable chairs. Storytime can take place in the book corner with the adult reading to a small group of children. Books and stories teach children to sit still for a short period of time, develop concentration, practise language and learn new words, experience emotions such as joy, excitement and fear, and share experiences with others, e.g. going to the dentist, getting a new brother or sister. Books are able to make the connections for the child between the symbol (picture) and the written word and the spoken word. Books are also informational, giving extra and exciting details about things seen on outings, in the shops, in the garden etc. The child's curiosity is stimulated to ask questions, and the adult can help the child to find answers from books.

The book corner should be in a quiet area of the room; it should be warm, well lit and comfortable. Books should be displayed attractively in a purpose-built display rack, which could be home-made. The books on display should be changed regularly. Many nurseries and schools have a system whereby children can take a book home overnight so they can read it with their parents. All the children must understand that the book corner is a quiet area of the room and that it is not the place for noisy or boisterous play. Children must be taught to handle books carefully and to respect them so that they can be shared by all the children. Any torn books should be mended straightaway, if possible making sure that the child who did the tearing is involved in the repairing. Old, tattered, dog-eared books should be removed as they will not be attractive to the children. Books should have pictures that reflect children from different cultures, different family styles and males and females in non-stereotypical roles. Books need to be very carefully chosen to ensure that they are not giving children the wrong messages about race, culture and equal opportunities.

Specialist suppliers like the Letter Box Library are able to provide lists of non-racist, non-sexist books for children (address in Appendix). Pop-up books are not suitable for group usage as they very easily get torn and look unattractive.

Traditional stories such as 'The Three Little Pigs', 'Billy Goats Gruff' and 'Tale of a Turnip' are popular, as they have a lot of repetition that the children like to join in. There are also translations of traditional Asian and Afro-Caribbean stories such as 'Anansi the

Spider' which are popular with children. Informational books should be colourful and have good clear illustrations. These books may become part of a display on the interest table. It is also useful to have a large picture encyclopaedia to enable the children to look up information about any topic they are particularly interested in.

When reading stories to children make sure that they are all sitting comfortably and that they can all see the book. Hold the book open and face the children as you read the story. Stop to point to illustrations or to ask the children questions. Read slowly and clearly with animation so that the children's interest is held. A good story-teller will be able to alter his voice to indicate excitement, fear, different characters in the story etc. It is essential for the adults to have read the story themselves before they read it to the children; this way they will become familiar with the story and be able to read it in a more animated way.

Storytelling was a custom long before books were written and was often a way of passing on oral history and information. A story can be told without a book but it may be a version of a story in a book or it can be a totally original story. Props such as puppets, bags and hats can be used to enliven the story. As in reading a story, the teller must adopt different voices for different characters and use her voice to express emotions. Telling stories well requires imagination and advance preparation on the part of the storyteller.

Children love rhymes and poetry as they enjoy the repetition and learn to join in. Action rhymes such as 'Miss Polly had a Dolly' are very popular, with children being able to play the different roles. Counting rhymes may help children to learn numbers, although much of this may be learning by rote as most of the rhymes require the child to count backwards! Stories told in rhyme have a great appeal to children, particularly if they are also ring games such as 'There was a Lovely Princess', which is the story of Sleeping Beauty in rhyme. The poems of AA Milne are very popular with older children (6–7 years) and may encourage children to write their own poetry. The basis of all poetry is the flow and rhythm of the language

SCENARIO 7.2

Your Officer-in-Charge has given you a budget of £200 to restock the book corner in your nursery room. The room caters for children between the ages of 3 and 4 years. Draw up a list of criteria that you will use in order to select the books.

SCENARIO 7.3

Gemma is 4 years old and at times is inclined to be disruptive. Today Gemma has torn three books in the book corner. How do you handle this situation so that Gemma develops a greater understanding of the way books should be treated?

used, described by Coleridge as 'the best words in the best order', therefore poems are a very early introduction to children of rhythm.

Music, Movement, Dance

Children can be introduced to musical sounds from a very early age; musical mobiles are available that can be suspended over the baby's cot. Children like to create their own musical sounds; even babies enjoy the tinkle of bells or the sound of the rattle. Adults sing to children and will play music to them from an early age. The lullaby is traditionally a calming quiet song that will soothe a baby. As children get older they can express their emotions through playing musical instruments or participating in music and movement. Music develops children's listening skills, trains their ear to distinguish between different musical instruments and introduces them to rhythms. Through music and movement sessions they are able to learn to control both large and small muscles, learn body coordination and move in time to the music. It also offers the opportunity for self-expression and creativity as they find a way to 'be a wave in a stormy sea' or 'be an elephant'. Most nurseries have a music area where different instruments are displayed. It is not necessary to purchase expensive instruments, as home-made shakers, bells, drums, tambourines, cymbals, gongs, recorders etc. will be all that is needed. Instruments from other cultures such as castanets, skin drums, pan pipes and bamboo pipes will broaden the children's knowledge and experience. Children can experiment with these, finding out what type of noise each makes and how they work, whether they are plucked, blown, shaken or banged. Children are able to clap out simple rhythmic patterns in songs, poems or music. Music can be used to calm feelings or express emotions; a good bang on a drum can release a lot of frustration.

Music also aids the development of children's listening skills. They have to learn to listen to music and other sounds around them. If you are going to clap in rhythm to the music then you must listen to the music. If you are going to sing accompanied by a piano or guitar then you must listen to the notes played on the instrument.

Children should be introduced to a wide variety of music using tapes. CDs or records; this is also an opportunity to play music from other cultures so that they get a broad view of what music is about. When children make their own music this can be tape-recorded and played back to them so they are able to listen to their own product.

Water Play

This can be an indoor or outdoor activity or could be helping the adult to wash up or wash clothes. The earliest form of water play for children is bath time. In the nursery there will be a purpose-made water trolley which is usually equipped with a large variety of pipes, tubes, sieves, plastic bottles, jugs, waterwheel, corks, wood, rock etc. Through their experimental and exploratory play with water, children learn about the properties of water, conservation of volume, sinking and floating, bubbles, and water as a source of power to turn a wheel. These are all early scientific concepts. If water play is outside on a hot summer day, they will also learn that the heat is able to dry spilt water and that the water gets warm in the heat. Water play is made more interesting by varying the equipment and colouring the water.

The child care worker needs to ask children questions which extend their understanding of the basic concepts and allow them to problem solve, for example, 'What happens if you fill one big jug with water, is there enough water to fill two small jugs?' 'Let's find out which of these toys sink and which float,' and 'What happens to water if it's put into the freezer?'

Playing with water can prove to be a very relaxing activity for children and adults. Water satisfies all the senses; it makes a lovely sound, it looks inviting and on a hot day a refreshing drink of clean cool water is welcomed. Water is a very versatile medium for children to use and they can repeat experiments over and over again. Most children like water: splashing in puddles, bath time, going to the paddling pool, watching ships and going to the seaside are pleasurable activities. There is a lot to find out about water, particularly when it is ice or snow. Water play can be a solitary activity or a cooperative activity, for example a group of children may decide to wash dolls' clothes and bath dolls, doing this together. Water play leads to a lot of communication between children and between adults and children.

Sand Play

Once again sand is a good medium for understanding scientific concepts such as flowing, gritty, moulding etc. Most nurseries and playgroups have a sand trolley. Sand play needs to offer children both wet and dry sand, as the concepts of each are different. Children like to bury things in sand and then rediscover these objects at a later point. Children can draw in wet sand and watch the picture disappear as the sand dries out; they can also draw a picture on paper using glue and then sprinkle dry sand over this.

As with water play, the role of the adult is one of extending the children's understanding and thinking and introducing them to the language which goes with the concepts. Questions can be asked such as 'What does dry sand feel like?' 'Which type of sand goes through the sieve the fastest, wet or dry?' and 'Are there any things which are the same about sand and water?'. Older children are able to make sand and water clocks to compare these likenesses and differences. Sand can be used indoors and outside; outside there is often a large sandpit which gives great scope for building large tunnels, castles and other structures. Sand play can be both a solitary activity and a cooperative activity. It does not have the same soothing effect upon children as water play, but it can prove to be just as exciting.

Playing with Clay Clay is another natural material that children like to play with. They will discover that it is more difficult to mould than dough and requires a lot of rolling, kneading and banging to get into shape. Children do not need a lot of equipment to play with clay, just a board and rolling pin; the rest they can do with their hands. Children's products can be kept and dried (there is clay available which does not need firing) and then the children can paint them.

Clay play is usually a solitary activity although children may be given a specific task such as moulding 'cakes' to go in the home corner or class shop, or making animals to go into the farm area, or forming three-dimensional shapes for maths. Because it needs a great deal of strength to mould, clay is not suitable for very young children; it is better to give them dough.

The role of the adult is very important in the storing of clay as it dries out very easily and is then unable to be used. Most nurseries will have a plastic clay bin which has a tight fitting lid; the clay is stored in this but first needs to be wrapped in a damp cloth and then placed in a plastic bag. Older children will be able to help the adult do this and understand the relationship between water and clay. Clay play is a very good medium for boisterous children to use in order to work out their aggression and excess energy.

Cooking/ Preparing Food

Older children love to participate in cooking or other food preparation activities. Cooking is a cooperative activity that is done in small groups and requires an adult to plan, lead and oversee the children to ensure safety. It is an excellent learning medium, starting with a visit to the shops to buy the required ingredients and ending with the children eating or taking home their products. Not all food activities require a cooker, for example making ice lollies, making sandwiches, making cold sweets by whisking substances into milk or making jellies.

From a cookery session, children will learn a great deal of science and maths: how heat changes substances, thickening through whisking, the effects of extreme cold on substances, weighing, counting different things in different ways e.g. eggs counted singly, flour weighed, flavourings in teaspoons or drops etc. Children will also learn how to listen to and carry out instructions, how to work together to weigh, mix, stir and knead, and how to share out the end product. They will also learn the beginnings of food hygiene, washing hands, cleaning the table, wearing an apron, how to treat knives with respect and cleaning up after themselves whilst the food is cooking. Different types of vegetables and fruit can be introduced and these can be explored by cutting them in half, peeling them and tasting them raw and cooked; children may even grow their own vegetables such as mustard and cress and then make sandwiches with them for lunch.

Language is developed by naming ingredients and utensils; and cooking terms (e.g. roll, knead, chop and grate); mathematical language (e.g. grammes, litres and kilos), and scientific language (e.g.

boiling, roasting, baking, melting and freezing), will all be explored in cookery. For some children who may live in a home where microwaved dinners are the norm, cooking can be a totally new experience. It is also a good time for the adult to talk to the children about healthy eating and to introduce foods from different cultures; this is an area where you may be able to involve parents in demonstrating different cooking utensils such as woks, paella pans etc.

Cooking is an all-round intensive learning situation, but is such an exciting activity that children are always more than willing to participate.

Interest Tables

Most nurseries and schools have an interest table which is changed on a regular basis. The interest table may be based on a particular theme, such as 'weather', 'cats' or 'mini-beasts', or maybe teaching children a particular concept, such as colours or numbers. The whole idea of an interest table is to bring together items that the children can examine, explore and discuss with the adult and with each other. It must look attractive; a few carefully chosen items are better than a packed table. All the items displayed must be safe for the children to touch and explore (no rough edges or sharp points, nothing toxic, precious or irreplaceable etc.). The staff team will usually decide on the themes for the interest table, and the staff may take it in turns to be responsible for themes. The interest table should also have informational books which are open at the appropriate pages, along with pictures, photographs or other illustrations. When the interest table is first set up, the children's attention should be drawn to it and it should be explained to them what it is about and how they can use it. This should be done each time that the theme is changed. Sometimes children will bring in additional items for the table and these should be put on display. Flowers and plants may be displayed and it is important to involve the children in watering and caring for them; however, children should be discouraged from picking flowers and plants to bring into school as they could be poisonous, and it is not in line with present thinking about conservation.

SETTING OUT AND CLEARING AWAY PLAY ACTIVITIES

It is the adult's responsibility to plan and organize play activities for children. The usual method of doing this is through a team meeting of all the staff who are working with the children. The school or nursery may have long term aims and objectives for the children and the adults will need to ensure that the activities enable the children to reach these aims. For example, the aim for the next month may be to encourage the children's concept development in maths and science and to extend their language and the theme may be 'the weather', therefore all activities for the next 2 weeks will start from the weather. In addition to this there may be specific learning goals for certain children who may have special needs or behaviour problems.

Planning

A weekly meeting of the team will decide on the activities and the specific responsibilities of each member of staff. Certain equipment is likely to be on hand every day for the children, such as water, sand, painting, dressing up, home corner etc.; however, it will probably be necessary to vary the equipment in each of these areas so that it fits in with the learning outcomes. For example, using the weather theme the dressing-up corner would have mackintoshes, umbrellas, scarves, hats, coats, gloves, sunshades, dark glasses etc.; the water trolley will have sprays, waterproof materials and ice; the cookery session will make hot things for cold days and cool drinks for hot days. Part of the planning may require some children going to the shops or on a small outing elsewhere. It is important to ensure that there is parental permission for this type of activity and the adults need to decide when they will go, who they will take, where they will go, what the purpose of the visit is and that there are enough adults to adequately supervise the number of children. Once the plans for the week have been made and all members of staff have been allocated their particular areas of responsibility, the plans should then be displayed on the inside of a cupboard door to ensure that everyone is aware of what everyone else is doing. This is particularly important if you are a candidate on placement as you may only be at the nursery for 2 days a week, but whatever you will be doing on those days needs to be communicated to all staff so that there is no duplication or confusion.

Setting Out Equipment

The adult's most important role in setting out activities is to ensure that they are in a position that is safe for the children. You may also need to consider access for children with special needs. Activities need to be kept well away from doors and main walkways.

The room should be set up well in advance of the children arriving. In many cases there is not a lot of alteration that can be done to the layout of the room. For example, the water trolley has a permanent spot close to the bathroom, the shop has replaced the home corner for a number of weeks, the quiet area/book corner is in a fixed position; the only features which may be open to movement are the tables. However, you can do quite a lot with tables, joining a number together for a large junk modelling activity or deciding whether the optimum number should be two or four children playing with the Lego etc. When putting out table toys it is important to think about the practicalities; if the Lego always ends up in the sand trolley then make sure that it is on a table as far away from the sand as possible. Remember the stages of development of the children and ensure that there are activities available that offer progressive complexity as well as those that are easy. There must be enough space for the children to walk easily around the tables and enough space on the tables for the number of participants to be able to play freely.

The equipment should look attractive to the children; this means no puzzles with missing pieces, attractive containers for Lego and Duplo, fresh paint and clean brushes, clean paper on the easels, clay that has not dried out, dressing-up clothes that are clean and displayed on hangers. Always make sure that you have protective aprons for water play, painting, clay and cooking, and allow the right number of aprons for the number of children participating in the activity. During the activities it is important to mop up any spillages quickly and ensure that there is always clean paper for painting, and fresh dough or clay when children change activity. Children should not have to reuse another child's leftover material; they should all have equal opportunity to use fresh materials.

Clearing Away Activities and Storing Equipment

Wherever possible the children should be involved in clearing away equipment as this is good training for them; however, this must be done in a safe way. Small equipment should be stored in clearly labelled boxes or trays on shelves or tray racks. Any products that the children wish to keep should be put in a safe place until home time. Paintings should be labelled with the child's name and pegged up to dry. Tables should be wiped down, dried and stacked in a safe place; do not get children to help in moving furniture. Jigsaws and matching games should be checked to ensure that all the pieces are complete. Paint pots should be cleaned or securely lidded if they are to be reused, and brushes must be washed and left to dry. Aprons must be washed and hung up to dry. Equipment should be regularly checked for safety and wear. Any equipment which needs mending should be removed from the play area and reported to the appropriate person. Outdoor equipment needs to be checked for rust and that nuts and bolts are not coming loose. Movable outdoor equipment should be kept in a locked shed, and sand pits should have a purpose-built cover to prevent cats and other animals polluting the sand.

EARLY YEARS CURRICULUM

The early years curriculum has been the subject of debate for many years and now few would deny that there is a range of learning opportunities offered to children in the pre-school years which can be defined in curriculum terms. Curtis (1986) stated, '... there is a recognizable curriculum for children under statutory school age based on skills and competencies to be developed in a flexible and child-centred environment, and there is ample material with which to challenge and extend children without offering them a "watered down" reception class programme.'

The Rumbold Committee (DES 1990) looked into the educational experiences offered to 3- and 4-year-olds, and in its report *Starting with Quality* defines the curriculum as follows:

> The curriculum – which we take to comprise the concepts, knowledge, understanding, attitudes and skills that a child needs to develop – can be defined and expressed in a number of different ways. These varying approaches include frameworks based on subjects, resource areas, broad themes or areas of learning.
>
> (DES 1990)

The Rumbold report gives the areas of learning which go towards constructing a curriculum for the under-fives as:

- Aesthetic and creative
- Human and social
- Language and literacy
- Mathematics
- Physical
- Science
- Spiritual and moral
- Technology.

Rumbold goes into great detail regarding the concepts and activities which come under each of these headings. However, the following is a concise version that is taken from a document produced by ILEA (1987):

> *Aesthetic and creative:* about symbolic representation, imaginative play, art and craft work, display, drama, movement and music. About doing their own creations and appreciating the creations of others.
>
> *Human and social:* about how we live and the world of work, about relationships with each other and the environment. About actions in the past and their relationship to the present and future. About physical and human conditions.
>
> *Language and literacy:* about symbolic representation and about listening, talking, reading and writing.
>
> *Mathematics:* about recognizing and solving problems, about sorting and classifying and identifying relationships and patterns.

About pure numbers, measures, logic and sets and their application to other areas.

Physical: about body awareness, coordination and control, about spatial, manipulative and motor skills. About imaginative use of the body, about health and its maintenance.

Scientific and technological: about problem solving, about changing and controlling the environment. About ourselves and living things, about physical surroundings, about forces, movement and energy.

Moral: about awareness of self and others, about right and wrong, fairness and justice. About being a member of a group and wider community.

Spiritual: about significance of life, about sense of awe and wonder, about myths and legends. About religious experiences reflecting many faiths.

(ILEA 1987)

There have been in existence for some time a number of curriculum models; some are based upon the theories of the well known educators upon whose philosophies they depend and others have developed for differing reasons. Five of these will be looked at in detail: Highscope, Steiner, Montessori, Portage and Early Learning Goals.

Highscope

This was first introduced in the USA in the 1960s as part of the Head Start programme. Head Start was a Federal initiative put into place to reduce the educational disadvantage of children from socially and economically deprived backgrounds. Highscope was introduced to the UK in the mid-1980s. Highscope programmes encourage children to be problem solvers and decision makers, and to attain independence through a framework of activities. Highscope places special emphasis on children planning their own activities and then reflecting upon how the activity went; this is known as Plan–Do–Review. A typical Highscope day would be broken into: greeting, planning time, work time, clean up time, recall time, circle time, small group time, outside time, end of session and recording, when the adults write up their account of each child. Highscope materials clearly define what each child should be doing and also what each adult's role should be during the activity. From this point of view the Highscope method is highly structured.

Rudolf Steiner (1861–1925)

The methods based upon the philosophy of Steiner are ref[
the Waldorf education system. Steiner believed that childho
as a period of life in its own right and he was concerned ab
oping all the characteristics of the growing child. The Waldorf curriculum aims to give the child a balanced experience of arts and
sciences and balance in the processes of thinking, feeling and willing.
It seeks to educate more than just the intellect, giving the child open
options to learn. The environment of the nursery is very important and
must provide a warm joyful atmosphere. The day may begin with a
circle activity and singing games. Children are free to play with others
or alone. Play is usually with natural materials; there are no manufactured toys or games. There are seasonal decorations such as leaves,
twigs, pine cones, stones, crystals, rocks etc. There are numerous
wooden blocks of different sizes, textures and shapes. Imaginative
play is a central activity in the Waldorf system. The role of the teacher
is to be ready to help or join in. The teacher is leader, instigator and
role model as she has the task of firing the children's imaginations by
telling stories (not reading stories), singing songs, playing games,
pointing out things in the natural world, painting alongside the children, baking, sewing etc. The teacher must be well prepared and a
good role model for the children to imitate.

Maria Montessori (1869–1952)

Montessori's philosophy is based upon enabling each child to
develop to its full potential. She believed that children's minds are
able to absorb complex concepts about the world around them in
an effortless way. She saw children learning through observation,
exploration and movement. Montessori nursery schools are meant to
be a homely environment with different areas for quiet activities,
table work, floor activities and free access to a garden. Children
have the freedom to choose what they wish to do and spend as long
as they need on an activity. Independence and self-motivation are
encouraged. Children work with specially designed equipment
which enables them to make discoveries about the world around
them. The adult's role is to involve himself by working alongside the
child, to prepare the environment to enable children to learn spontaneously, to act as a link between the child and the materials and
to observe the children. As the adults observe the children they take
notes and decide which materials should be presented next in order
for the children to progress to the next development stage.

Portage

This is a system which was devised in the USA. It is a structured
home-based programme to teach children skills and is most useful

for children with special needs or developmental delay. Portage is delivered by specially trained people who may be teachers, health workers or volunteers. The Portage worker negotiates with parents and carers as to which skills will be taught to the child. The parents and carers are responsible for repeating the programme with the child between the visits of the Portage worker and for recording the progress of the child. The Portage package consists of teaching cards, activity charts and checklists which cover infant stimulation, socialization, and self-help, language, cognitive and motor skills. It is a very highly structured system with each task broken down into

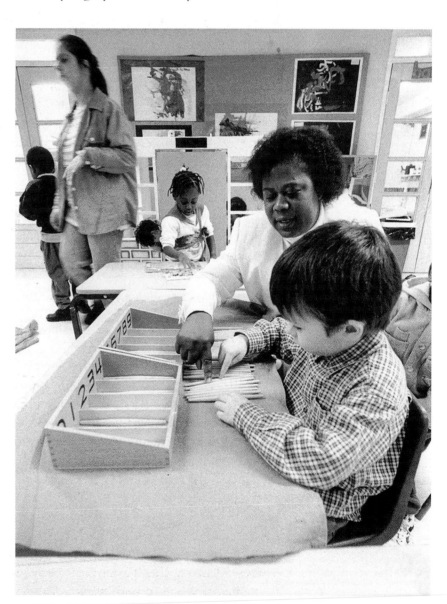

small steps, each step being slightly more complex than the preceding step. Because it is very structured it works best with parents and carers who are highly motivated and well organized. Although the aim of the Portage system is predominantly to benefit the child, it often leads to parents and carers having a better understanding of the child and helps them to develop more confidence in working with the child.

Early Learning Goals

The curriculum for the Early Learning Goals consists of the following ten areas for children.

Personal, social and emotional wellbeing: in particular by supporting the transition to and between settings, promoting an inclusive ethos and providing opportunities for each child to become a valued member of that group and community so that a strong self-image and self-esteem are promoted.

Positive attitudes and dispositions towards their learning: in particular an enthusiasm for knowledge and learning, and a confidence in their ability to be successful learners.

Social skills: in particular by providing opportunities that enable them to learn how to cooperate and work harmoniously alongside, and with, each other and to listen to each other.

Attention skills and persistence: in particular the capacity to concentrate on their own play or on group tasks.

Language and communication: with opportunities for all children to talk and communicate in a widening range of situations, to respond to adults and to each other, to practise and extend the range of vocabulary and communication skills they use and to listen carefully.

Reading and writing: with opportunities for all children to explore, enjoy, learn about, and use words and text in a broad range of contexts and to experience a rich variety of books.

Mathematics: with opportunities for all children to develop their understanding of number, measurement, pattern, shape and space by providing a broad range of contexts in which they can explore, enjoy, learn, practise and talk about them.

Knowledge and understanding of the world: with opportunities for all children to solve problems, make decisions, experiment, predict, plan and question in a varied range of contexts;

and to explore and find out about their environment and people and places that have significance in their lives.

Physical development: with opportunities for all children to develop and practise their fine and gross motor skills, increase their understanding of how their bodies work and what they need to be healthy and safe.

Creative development: with opportunities for all children to explore and share their thoughts, ideas and feelings through a variety of art, design and technology, music, movement, dance and imaginative and role-play activities.

(QCA 1999)

What the child should have achieved by the end of the foundation stage (i.e. by the age of 5 years) is clearly stated in the documentation produced by QCA. An example of these goals is as follows:

Early Learning Goals for Physical Development. By the end of the foundation stage, most children will be able to:

- Move with confidence, imagination and in safety
- Move with control and coordination
- Show awareness of space, of themselves and of others
- Recognize the importance of keeping healthy and those things which contribute to this
- Recognize the changes that happen to their bodies when they are active
- Use a range of small and large equipment
- Travel around, under, over and through balancing and climbing equipment
- Handle tools, objects, construction and malleable materials safely and with increasing control.

(QCA 1999)

OBSERVATION AND ASSESSMENT C4

A feature of all early years curricula is that there should be an element of observation and assessment of the child in order to record the child's progress. Information on the abilities of the child is useful for the parents, the school and the child's developmental records. Teachers and child care workers are able to plan a programme of future activities for children if they are aware of the developmental stages the children have reached and the competences that they already have. Certain children may need extra help or may need to spend longer on specific activities. The responsibility for undertaking and recording assessment usually lies with the teacher, the nursery officer or the most senior person working with a group of children. However, all staff are able to make contributions by carrying out observations on groups of children or target children. Observing children is a basic skill needed by all those who are intending to work with children. It is a skill that can be developed through training and practised 'on the job'. Confidentiality is an important aspect of observation and assessment, and any observations which are going to be used for purposes outside of the placement must ensure that the child remains anonymous or that the parents or guardians have given permission for the observation to be used.

Baseline Assessment

This national framework has been devised to assess children when they enter primary school at aged 5.3 years. Baseline assessment is intended to provide information to teachers so that they can plan effectively to meet individual children's learning needs and measure children's attainment in order to plot their progress. The Qualifications and Curriculum Authority (QCA) have produced assessment instruments and all maintained schools are required to use these in order to carry out the baseline assessment process. It is expected that the Early Learning Goals will help children towards getting good scores at the point of baseline assessment.

National Literacy Strategy

In order to improve the literacy skills of all children the government has introduced the National Literacy Strategy. Since September 1999 all primary schools must implement the literacy hour. This involves an hour of the timetable when the whole class shares a book together and undertakes some reading and writing. There is teacher directed work and independent work. For 75% of the literacy hour the whole class is taught by the teacher either in small groups or as a whole group. The framework for the Strategy provides a structured term-by-term guide on what should be taught during the literacy hour.

National Numeracy Strategy

Since September 1999 all schools have had a daily numeracy hour based on very similar lines to the literacy hour. The framework for the Strategy provides the structure for the numeracy hour and offers a term-by-term guide on what should be taught. Whilst the majority of the time is spent on teacher-led whole group activities, there is also the opportunity for children to work in small groups or independently.

ASSIGNMENTS

1. Write an essay on the value of play for the child.

2. Describe a typical water play session and describe which Early Learning Goals the activity would cover.

3. Write an essay on what you understand by the term 'inclusion'.

4. Describe the role and responsibilities of the adult in relation to children's play.

5. What do you understand by the National Literacy and Numeracy Strategies? How will these benefit children?

PRACTICAL ACTIVITIES

1. Draw a plan of a nursery room showing the layout of activities that will be available for the children. Give reasons for your choice of layout.

2. Write a plan for a cookery session for a group of six 3-year-olds. Give full explanations of the choice of recipe, how you will organize the session and what you expect the children to learn from the session.

3. Undertake the following observations and evaluate each observation in the light of your knowledge of child development and learning:
   a. A $2\frac{1}{2}$-year-old playing with dry sand
   b. A 3-year-old playing in the dressing-up corner
   c. A music and movement session for a group of 4-year-olds
   d. A 5-year-old painting.

4. Draw up a programme of activities for a group of 4-year-olds around the theme of pets. Explain what the children will learn from each activity and identify the Early Learning Goals that each activity will cover.

References

Athey C 1990 Extending thought in young children: a parent teacher partnership. Paul Chapman, London

Bee H 1992 The developing child, p323. Harper Collins, New York

Brierley J 1987 Give me a child until he is seven: brain studies and early childhood education. Falmer Press, London

Curtis A 1986 A curriculum for the pre-school child: learning to learn. NFER-Nelson, Windsor

Department of Health 1993 The rights of the child: a guide to the UN convention. HMSO, London

DES 1990 Starting with quality: report of the committee of inquiry into the quality of the educational experience offered to 3–4 years olds. HMSO, London

ILEA 1987 The early years: a curriculum for young children. ILEA Learning Resources Branch, London

Isaacs S 1954 The educational value of the nursery school. British Association for Early Childhood Education, London (still available from BAECE)

Jameson K 1973 Pre-school and infant art. Studio Vista, London

Kellogg R 1955 What children scribble and why. National Press, California

Qualifications and Curriculum Authority/DFEE 1999 Early learning goals. QCA, London

Further reading

■ Britton L 1992 Montessori play and learn. Vermilion, London

■ Bruce T 1989 Early childhood education. Hodder & Stoughton, Sevenoaks

■ Bruce T 1991 Time to play in early childhood education. Hodder & Stoughton, Sevenoaks

■ Buddulph L, McQueen D 1995 How to help talking. First Community Health NHS Trust, Cannock, Staffs.

■ David T 1992 Curriculum in the early years. In: Pugh G (ed) Contemporary issues in the early years. NCB/Paul Chapman, London

■ Derman-Sparks L 1989 Anti-bias curriculum: tools for empowering young children. National Association for the Education of Young Children, Washington DC

■ Drummond MJ, Lally M, Pugh G 1989 Developing a curriculum for the early years. National Children's Bureau, London

■ Drummond MJ, Nutbrown C 1992 Observing and assessing young children. In: Pugh G (ed) Contemporary issues in the early years. NCB/Paul Chapman, London

■ Hurst V 1991 Planning for early learning: education in the first 5 years. Paul Chapman, London

■ Lindstrom M 1957 Children's art. University of California Press, California

■ Matterson E 1989 Play with a purpose for the under sevens, 3rd edn. Penguin, London

■ Nutbrown C 1994 Threads of thinking: young children learning and the role of early education. Paul Chapman, London

■ Nutbrown C 1996 Children's rights and early education. Paul Chapman, London

■ Pugh G, De'Ath E 1989 Working towards partnership in the early years. National Children's Bureau, London

Chapter 8

Working with Parents and Primary Carers

This chapter covers underpinning knowledge for parts of the following units for the National Vocational Qualifications (NVQs) in Early Years Care and Education: P1, P4, P5, P8, P9. This chapter is also linked to the following CACHE Awards Units: Diploma Unit 11; Certificate Unit Option B.

INTRODUCTION

This chapter will explore the professional relationship which all child care workers need to create with a child's parents or primary carers. We live in a society that has the highest divorce rate in Europe and as a consequence of this many children may live with only one parent, with step-parents or with primary carers who may be grandparents, aunts, an older sibling, foster carers etc. However, it is most important that the child care worker respects that the parent or primary carer at this moment in time is the most important person in the child's life, and is the person responsible for the child's day-to-day welfare and development. Child care workers must not be judgmental about the way parents or primary carers are performing in this role. Most parents strive to do their best in an area that they may have no training in or very little knowledge about. Parenting is a very difficult task and nobody ever gets it totally right, whatever textbooks may lead you to believe! You must always remember that the child will love its parents or primary carers even if they appear to be very inadequate parents, and it is every child care worker's responsibility to empower and enable them to become better parents. Many parents and carers may have low self-esteem because of their own family background or because of a failed marriage or other negative experiences which they have had. Many lone parents may feel very isolated and may have become unused to socializing and making new friends. The day care setting is an ideal place to offer facilities for parent and carers as well as for the children. A recent government initiative has been the designation of some child care centres as Early Excellence Centres. These centres, in addition to providing a full day care and out of school service, are also able to be a 'one stop shop' offering help and advice for parents, including adult education classes. Wherever possible, other early years establishments should be working towards offering advice and becoming a 'one stop shop' for parents.

PARENTS AS PARTNERS

The DFEE (1996a,b) highlights the very influential role that parents/ primary carers have upon the learning achievements of the child. The home experiences of the child are significant and will be reflected in the child's learning at nursery or school. It is therefore important that child care workers acknowledge this influence and work in partnership with parents. Braun (1992) points out that there is a failure on the part of child care workers to recognize just how much parents achieve for their children; this failure is seen through the negative attitudes which many workers have towards parents. Braun (1992) believes that most parents have the highest aspirations for their children, although they may lack the necessary information and resources to meet these aspirations. Involving parents in their children's care and education will give them confidence and this has very positive spin-offs for the child.

> **SCENARIO** 8.1
>
> Chen Lee is 4 years old and has just started at your nursery school. On his first day at school his mother, Mrs Chen, was very reluctant to stay with him. Draw up a programme of how you could best make a relationship with Mrs Chen and encourage her to participate in her son's learning.

Pugh and De'Ath (1989) put forward 10 key factors that can help or hinder partnerships with parents and about which the establishment must make decisions and implement policies. Braun (1992) offers a shorter list of ways in which parents and families can be involved:

(1) there might be space set aside, such as a parents' room where parents can meet or drop in for a chat to one another;
(2) parents or other family members might be used as helpers – in regular group activities, or less regularly, on trips;
(3) specific provision might be made, e.g. parent and toddler group or parenting groups aimed to support parents in their role;
(4) particular attention might be focused on communications at the beginning and end of a session, when families are leaving and then collecting children;

(5) parents can be involved in the management of the service, through membership of its governing body or management committee.

(Braun 1992)

Parents must be made to feel welcome and there should be opportunities for them to participate in activities, exchange information with the child care workers, meet other parents and be informed of their child's progress. They should also be given information about the curriculum and ways in which they can help their child. Parents from ethnic groups may like to be invited to tell the children stories, rhymes or music from their culture or explain about their foods and demonstrate ethnic cooking utensils. Some parents may find it difficult to become involved in this way as they may be working or studying full time, may feel embarrassed or be shy, or they may not feel that they have an adequate command of English if this is not their first language. Braun (1992) points out that child care staff often confuse a parent's non-involvement with disinterest rather than taking time to find the real reasons. The first starting point in forming a relationship is to have respect for parents, listen to what they have to say and not to make assumptions about people.

Relationships should be developed remembering that they are important for the child, whose welfare is paramount, for the parent and for the child care worker. Staff should not let their own attitudes and values exert an influence on relationships with parents. Many establishments have a particular member of staff who is responsible for liaison with parents; this person may have had training in dealing with parents and needs to be a very good communicator. Parents have a right to know the mission statement of the establishment, the content of the curriculum and how they will be informed of their children's progress before they make a decision to send them to that nursery, playgroup or school. Parents would wish to know that the

SCENARIO 8.2

Mrs Fitzgerald is the primary carer for her 3-year-old granddaughter Siobhan. Mrs Fitzgerald is very reluctant even to enter the nursery when she drops Siobhan off. The Nursery Officer has had a chat with Mrs Fitzgerald who has expressed her lack of self confidence in actively participating in the activities of the nursery. Draw up a strategy which would help Mrs Fitzgerald overcome her fears and help her actively to participate.

establishment that their child will attend will not be in conflict with their own values, religion or culture.

Many nurseries and schools now have a policy relating to Parents as Partners. The policy covers areas such as open access to children's records, representation on management committees, open access to the nursery premises and how to make suggestions on nursery matters.

INVOLVING PARENTS/ CARERS

It is important that parents/carers are involved in their child's day-to-day activities in the setting. Usually a member of the senior staff is responsible for the liaison with parents; however, individual nursery officers or teachers may chat to parents/carers about the daily progress of the child. Whilst junior members of staff and students would not be expected to undertake a direct liaison role with parents, it is expected that they would be welcoming to them and able to direct them to the appropriate person who can give them the information they need.

Parents/carers need to be actively encouraged to participate in the activities of the setting. This may be difficult for parents who are working as they may not have the time to visit during the session; however, it is still important to keep them informed as they may have time off during the day which would enable them to spend a few hours in the nursery. When parents/carers collect their children from the setting it is important that they are given feedback on the positive things that the child has achieved during the day. It is very demoralizing to be told about all the wrong things that the child has done or how badly the child has behaved. This type of feedback can result in parents feeling guilty about leaving their child or feeling that the nursery is against their child. Daily feedback is particularly important for those who are parents/carers of babies, as they progress and develop rapidly and everyone needs to be aware of what stage of development the child has reached.

Some settings have organized parent sessions which enable parents and carers to network with each other and to make their expectations clear to the staff. It is also an opportunity to offer information on particular topics by visiting speakers addressing the meeting. This is especially useful when there are particular areas of concern such as the outbreak of an infectious illness e.g. chicken-pox, or national fears about an illness such as meningitis. Parents/carers are able to bring their skills or talents to the nursery and may visit specifically to undertake a particular session with the children, such as woodwork, ethnic cooking, dancing, music or story telling.

Sharing these skills and talents with the children enables parents to feel positive and confident about their role in relation to the setting and helps to build up positive relationships between parents and staff. It is also good for the children's self-esteem to see their parents/carers participating in the nursery alongside the staff.

CONFIDENTIALITY   If parents are to trust staff in the nursery it is important that staff are aware of the importance of confidentiality. Most establishments operate on a 'need to know' basis whereby confidential information is only imparted by the senior staff to those who need to know it in order to ensure the welfare of the child. Students and trainees are first introduced to the importance of confidentiality when they are recording information about children or undertaking child observations. It must not be possible to identify a child from a case study or observation. If a student or trainee wants to include photographs in a portfolio he must have the parent's permission in writing in order to do this. Confidentiality about children and their families is one of the most important aspects of child care work. Sometimes parents will find themselves relating to a particular student/trainee and may begin to disclose confidential information to them. It is important that the student respects this information as confidential and also talks to a senior member of staff about the situation. It must be remembered that as a junior member of staff you are unlikely to have the skills and information to offer the right sort of help to the parent. Whilst 'listening' is an important skill, it is just as important to be able to recognize what you should do with the information you have been given. It is not in the role of junior staff members to make these types of decisions but it is within their role to refer the information to the relevant staff member. It is important that trainees are aware of the boundaries and scope of their role and the lines of management and reporting.

SCENARIO 8.3

You are a trainee in a nursery in the Red Room. Ms Cooper, who is Angela's mother, seems very distressed and starts to tell you what is happening between her and her estranged partner, Angela's father. How do you handle this and what do you say to Ms Cooper?

COMMUNICATION WITH PARENTS/ CARERS

One of the most important skills that needs to be developed by the child care worker is how to communicate with parents/carers, children, fellow workers and professionals from outside agencies. Good communication skills are essential for the child care worker's role. Communicating with parents and carers can be a tricky process as they may have their own agendas which they are working to and which are not necessarily the same as yours. For example, you may be trying to communicate to Mrs A why it is important for her to bring her child to the nursery at a reasonable hour every day (your agenda), whereas Mrs A sees the nursery as trying to control her life by getting at her through her child (Mrs A's agenda). This type of situation can lead to very difficult communications in which no party benefits from the transaction. Parents such as Mrs A need very careful handling and need experienced communicators to deal with them. Wherever possible parents and carers need to be communicated with clearly, positively and honestly. It is not the role of the nursery worker to make parents feel guilty, disapproved of or threatened. Therefore all communication should be on a positive note, telling them the good things that the nursery can offer to them and their child and respecting their opinions and feelings.

The main ways that we communicate are verbally or in writing. However, during conversation there may also be a great deal of communication going on via body language and this may sometimes differ from the spoken message. Body language is communicated via facial expression, eye contact, position of the body etc. and it can be positive or negative. Examples of positive body language are good eye contact, an assuring tone of voice, leaning towards the speaker etc. Examples of negative body language are not making eye contact with the speaker, looking bored, yawning, day dreaming etc.

All communication needs to be clear, using simple easily understood language whilst not sounding patronizing. The object of any communication is to give and receive messages, information or advice. It is always useful, after you have explained something, to ask the question 'Have I explained that satisfactorily?' This allows the parent or carer the opportunity to mention those areas that they do not understand without them having to ask. Listening is an important part of the communication process and you need to let the other person know that you have been listening to them. The easiest way to do this is by summing up for them what you understand they have said, but start this by saying, 'Am I right in saying that you …'. This method also ensures that you have not misinterpreted the message.

In some instances where a parent or carer may come from an ethnic group they may not have a good command of the English language. If there are serious difficulties in communication it is useful to try to arrange for an interpreter to be present at the next meeting. The interpreter may be another member of the family who has been chosen by the parent or carer to accompany them. However, it is not good practice to suggest using the older children in the family as interpreters as this can be embarrassing for the carer and the content of the conversation may be totally inappropriate for an older child to be dealing with. In some areas the local authority is able to provide free interpretation services.

Written communication should be clear and to the point. If handwritten, the writing should be easily legible; if you have handwriting which is difficult to read then it is better to type or word process written communications. If the establishment is in an area where there are groups that have English as an additional language then translations of written communications are one way of ensuring that the message reaches the carers. The tone of the communication should be one of mutual respect and should not appear as patronizing.

PARENTAL ATTITUDES, EXPECTATIONS AND ROLES

Parents, like child care workers, come from a variety of social backgrounds. Just as with children, no two parents are the same. This means that they, like the children, must be treated as individuals. There is often an assumption, when referring to parental involvement, that all parents will leap at the opportunity to be involved in the establishment their child is attending. This is not always the case and there may be many reasons for their lack of enthusiasm in this direction. Some parents may feel guilty about leaving their child while they go to work, others may feel guilty because social services have found them the nursery place in order to ensure their child's needs are met. Other parents may be the opposite of those described above and may be over-enthusiastic in their involvement with the nursery. These may be the professionals, who are paying high fees for their children to be cared for and as a consequence see it as their duty to ensure that the nursery is keeping its part of the bargain. These parents may have high expectations, see themselves as customers, and demand to exert their authority. Whichever end of the spectrum parents are coming from, the child care worker must maintain respect for them as they are the child's primary carers. The nursery needs to steer a middle path and senior management is responsible for ensuring that all staff are aware of what this involves.

As important as their attitudes to the nursery will be the parents' attitudes to their children. Again this may range from those who are lacking in any interest in their child through to those who have very high expectations of their child. Neither of these extremes takes into account the stage of development and actual abilities of the child. It is important that the nursery shares with parents the developmental progress of their child so that they are aware of what their child can do. Many nurseries have a parental involvement policy, which ensures parents are able to review their child's progress on a regular basis. From these regular reviews it is hoped that parents will have a realistic view of what they can expect from their child. Some parents may need encouragement to meet with staff in order to review their child's progress, perhaps because they fear a negative report. It is important that child care workers emphasize what children can do, rather than giving parents a catalogue of what the child cannot do.

Some parents may be unsure of exactly what their role is in relation to the nursery. Maybe they think that it is like school: they drop their child at the door and come back to collect them by waiting outside in the playground. This image may be based on the way things were when they went to school themselves. They may think that being invited on outings is a courtesy gesture and they are not really expected to attend. In some cases, parents may think that any involvement in the nursery may lead to staff judging their performance as a parent. The nursery needs to explain to parents the benefits of their involvement, both for their children and for themselves. It is also important to explain to parents what their role is in relation to attending nursery outings, helping with activities etc. It is important that parents are not made to feel pressurized into taking on roles they do not feel comfortable with, and they should not feel that the staff are making demands upon them. However, it is also, important to emphasize what parents might expect to get out of participating in these activities, since possibly the most important aspect of parental involvement is the role of parents as sharers of their child's experiences.

ASSIGNMENTS

1. Write an essay on the reasons why parental involvement is important for children in day care setting.

2. What factors may influence a parent/carer's attitude to becoming involved in the day care setting that their child attends?

3. How can the day care setting encourage parental involvement?

4. Write an essay explaining how effective communication between the day care setting and the parent/carer can be achieved.

PRACTICAL ACTIVITIES

1. Make a list of all the policies in your day care setting, which might be of interest to parents.

2. Write a model Parental Involvement Policy.

3. Interview 4 parents from different backgrounds and ask them about the benefits they get from being involved in their child's day care establishment. Write up your answers and draw conclusions.

4. Draw up a strategy for how you will involve parents in the next nursery outing to the local zoo.

References

Braun D 1992 Working with parents. In: Pugh G (ed) Contemporary issues in the early years. National Children's Bureau, London

DFEE 1996a Nursery education scheme: the next steps. HMSO, London

DFEE 1996b Nursery education: desirable outcomes for children's learning on entering compulsory education. HMSO, London

Pugh G, De'Ath E 1989 Working towards partnership in the early years. National Children's Bureau, London

Further reading

■ Hay S 1997 Essential nursery management. Baillière Tindall, London

■ Pugh G, De'Ath E, Smith C 1994 Confident parents, confident children. National Children's Bureau, London

■ Rennie J 1996 Working with parents. In: Pugh G (ed) Contemporary issues in the early years, 2nd edn. National Children's Bureau, London

■ Sadek E, Sadek J 1996 Good practice in nursery management. Stanley Thornes, Cheltenham, UK

Useful Addresses

Action for Sick Children	First Floor, 300 Kingston Road, London, SW20 8LX Tel: 020 8542 4848 Fax: 020 8542 2424 www.actionforsickchildren.org
Advisory Centre for Education (ACE)	Unit 1B, Aberdeen Studios, 22 Highbury Grove, London, N5 2DQ Tel: 020 7354 8321
Advisory Council for the Education of Romany and Other Travellers (ACERT)	Moot House, The Stow, Harlow, Essex, CM20 3AG Tel: 01279 418 666
Afro-Caribbean Education Resource Project (ACER)	Acer Centre, Wyvil School, Wyvil Road, London, SW8 2TJ Tel: 020 627 2662 Fax: 020 7627 0278
Anti Bullying Campaign (ABC)	185 Tower Bridge Road, London, SE1 2UF Tel: 020 7378 1446 Fax: 020 7378 8374
Association for Brain Damaged Children and Young Adults	Clifton House, 3 St Paul's Road, Foleshill, Coventry, CV6 5DE Tel: 01203 665 450 abdcya@care4free.net
Association for Post Natal Illness (APNI)	25 Jerdon Place, London, SW6 1BE Tel: 020 7386 0868 Fax: 020 7386 8885 www.apni.org
Association for Spina Bifida and Hydrocephalus (ASBAH)	ASBAH House, 42 Park Road, Peterborough, PE1 2UQ Tel: 01733 555 988 Fax: 01733 555 985 www.asbah.demon.co.uk

Association of Breastfeeding Mothers (ABM)	PO Box 441, St Albans, Hertfordshire, AL4 0AS Tel: 020 7813 1481
Association of Parents of Vaccine Damaged Children	78 Camden Road, Shipston on Stour, Warwickshire, CV36 4DH Tel: 01608 667 959
BACUP	3 Bath Place, Rivington Street, London EC2A 3DR Tel: 020 7696 9003 Fax: 020 7696 9002 www.cancerbacup.org.uk
Birth Defects Foundation (BDF)	Chelsea House, Westgate, London, W12 1DR Tel: 01543 462 777 Fax: 01543 468 999 www.birthdefects.co.uk
Black Childcare Network	17 Brownhill Road, Catford, London, SE6
BLISS (National Charity of the New Born)	2nd Floor, 89 Albert Embankment, Camelford House, London, SE1 7TP Tel: 020 7820 9471 Fax: 020 7820 9567 www.bliss.org.uk
British Association for Early Childhood Education (BAECE)	136 Cavell Street, London, E1 2JA Tel: 020 7539 5400 Fax: 020 7539 5409 www.early-education.org.uk
British Association for the Study and Prevention of Child Abuse and Neglect (BASPCAN)	10 Priory Street, York, YO1 1EZ Tel: 01904 613 605 Fax: 01904 642 239 www.baspcan.org.uk
British Diabetic Association	10 Queen Anne St, London W1G 9LH Tel: 020 7323 1531 Fax: 020 7637 3644 www.diabetes.org.uk
Brittle Bone Society	30 Guthrie Street, Dundee DD1 5BS Tel: 01382 204446 Fax: 01382 206771 www.brittlebone.org.uk
Campaign for State Education (CASE)	158, Durham Road, London, SW20 0DG Tel: 020 8944 8206
Centre for Young Children's Rights	356 Holloway Road, London, N7 6PA Tel: 020 7700 8127 Fax: 020 7697 0982 www.scfuk.org.uk

Child Accident Prevention Trust (CAPT)	4th Floor, 18–20 Farringdon Lane, London, EC1R 3HA Tel: 020 7608 3828 Fax: 0207 608 3674
The Child Bereavement Trust	Aston House, High Street, West Wycombe, High Wycombe, Buckinghamshire, HP14 3AG Tel: 01494 446 648 Fax: 01494 440 057 www.childbereavement.org.uk
Child Growth Foundation	2 Mayfield Avenue, Chiswick, London, W4 1PW Tel: 020 8995 0257/8994 7625 Fax: 020 8995 9075 www.cgf.org.uk
Child Poverty Action Group (CPAG)	94 White Lion Street, London, N1 9PF Tel: 020 7837 7979 Fax: 020 7837 6414 www.cpag.org.uk
Childline	2nd Floor, Royal Mail Buildings, Studd Street, London, N1 0QW Tel: 020 7239 1000 Fax: 020 7239 1001 www.childline.org.uk
Childline Cymru	9th Floor, Alexandra House, Alexandra Road, Swansea, SA1 5ED Tel: 01792 480 111 Fax: 01792 480 333 www.childline.org.uk
Childrens 1st: Royal Scottish Society for Prevention of Cruelty to Children (RSSPCC)	Melville House, 41 Polwarth Terrace, Edinburgh EH11 1NU Tel: 0131 337 8539 Fax: 0131 446 8284
Childrens Rights Development Unit	235 Shaftsbury Avenue, London WC2H 8EL Tel: 020 7240 4449 Fax: 020 7240 4514
Commission for Racial Equality (CRE)	Elliot House, 10–12 Allington Street, London SW1E 5EH Tel: 020 7828 7022 Fax: 020 7630 7605 www.cre.gov.uk
Council for Awards in Children's Care and Education (CACHE)	8 Chequer Street, St Albans, Hertfordshire, AL1 3XZ Tel: 01727 847 636 Fax: 01727 867 609 www.cache.org.uk
Council for Disabled Children (CDC)	National Children's Bureau, 8 Wakeley Street, London, EC1V 7QE Tel: 020 7843 6000 Fax: 020 7278 9572 www.ncb.org.uk

The Countryside Agency	19 Dacre Street, London SW1H 0DH Tel: 020 7340 2900 www.countryside.gov.uk
Cruse Bereavement Care	Cruse House, 126 Sheen Road, Richmond, Surrey, TW9 1UR Tel: 020 8940 4818 Fax: 020 8940 7638 Bereavement line: 0845 758 5565
CRY-SIS Support Group	BM CRY-SIS, London, WC1N 3XX Tel: 020 7404 5011
Disablement Information and Advice Lines (DIAL UK)	St Catherines, Tickhill Road, Doncaster, DN4 8QN Tel: 01302 310 123 Fax: 01302 310 404 www.members.aol.com/dialuk
Down's Syndrome Association (DSA)	155 Mitcham Road, London, SW17 9PG Tel: 020 8682 4001 Fax: 020 8682 4012 www.downs-syndrome.org.uk
Early Years Trainers Anti-Racist Network (EYTARN)	PO Box 28, Wallasey, CH45 9NP Tel: 0151 639 6136
End Physical Punishment of Children (EPOCH)	77 Holloway Road, London, N7 8JZ Tel: 020 7700 0627 Fax: 020 7700 1105
Enuresis Resource and Information Centre (ERIC)	34 Old School House, Brittania Road, Kingswood, Bristol, BS15 8DB Tel: 0117 960 3060 Fax: 0117 960 0401 www.eric.org.uk
Equal Opportunities Commission (EOC)	Arndale House, Arndale Centre, Manchester, M4 3EQ Tel: 0161 833 9244 Fax: 0161 838 8312 www.eoc.org.uk
Exploring Parenthood	20a Treadgold Street, London W11 4BP Tel: 020 7221 4471 Fax: 020 7221 501
Family Nurturing Network	Ground Floor, Temple Court, 109 Oxford Road, Cowley, Oxford, OX4 2ER Tel: 01865 777756 Fax: 01865 777702 www.fnn.org.uk
Family Welfare Association (FWA)	501–505 Kingsland Road, Dalston, London, E8 4AU Tel: 020 7254 6251 Fax: 020 7249 5443 fwa.headoffice@fwa.org.uk

Foundation for the Study of Infant Deaths (FSID)

Artillery House, 11–19 Artillery Road, London, SW1P 1RT
Tel: 020 7222 8001   Fax: 020 7222 8002   www.sids.org.uk/fsid

Gingerbread

16–17 Clerkenwell Close, London EC1A 0AN
Tel: 020 7366 8183   Fax: 020 7336 8185   www.gingerbread.org.uk

Gingerbread Northern Ireland

169 University Street, Belfast, BT7 1HR, Northern Ireland
Tel: 028 90 231 568   www.gingerbreadni.org

Grandparents' Federation

Room 3, Moat House, The Stow, Harlow, Essex, CN20 3AG
Tel: 01279 444 964

Hartley-Brewer Parenting

117 Corringham Road, London, NE11 7DL
Tel: 020 8458 8404   www.cooperativekids.com

High/Scope UK

Copperfield House, 190–192 Maple Road, London, SE20 8HT
Tel: 020 8676 0220   Fax: 020 8659 9938   www.high-scope.org.uk

Home-Start UK

2 Salisbury Road, Leicester, LE1 7QR
Tel: 0116 233 9955   Fax: 0116 233 0232   www.home-start.org.uk

Hyperactive Children's Support Group (HACSG)

71 Whyke Lane, Chichester, West Sussex, PO19 2LD
Tel: 01903 752 182   Fax: 01903 734 726   www.hacsg.org.uk

Kid's Club Network

Bellerive House, 3 Muirfield Crescent, London, W14 9SZ
Tel: 020 7512 2112   Fax: 020 7512 2010   www.kidsclubs.com

Kidscape

2 Grosvenor Gardens, London, SW1W 0DH
Tel: 020 7730 3300   Fax: 020 7730 7081   www.kidscape.org.uk

La Leche League (Great Britain) (LLLGB)

BM 3424, London, WC1N 3XX
Tel: 020 7242 1278   www.stargate.co.uk/lllgb

Letterbox Library (Children's Books Ltd)

71–72 Allen Road, Hackney, London N16 8RY
Tel: 020 7503 4801   Fax: 020 7503 4800

Low Pay Unit

29 Amwell Street, London, W1Y 1TG
Tel: 020 7713 7616   Fax: 020 7713 7581   www.lowpayunit.org.uk

Meet-a-Mum Association (MAMA)	Waterside Centre, 26 Avenue Road, South Norwood, London, SE25 4DX Tel: 020 8771 5595 Fax: 020 8239 1153 www.MAMA.org.uk Helpline: 020 8768 0123
Mencap	123, Golden Lane, London, EC1Y 0RT Tel: 0207 454 0454 Fax: 0207 696 5540 www.mencap.org.uk
Meningitis Association Scotland	9 Edwin Street Glasgow, G51 1ND Tel: 0141 427 6698 (24 hour helpline) Fax: 0141 427 6698
Montessori Centre International	18 Balderton Street, London, W1Y 1TG Tel: 020 7493 0165 Fax: 020 7629 7808 www.montessori.ac.uk
Mudiad Ysgolion Meithrin (MYM)	145 Albany Street, Y Rhath, Caerdydd, CF24 3NT Tel: 029 2043 6800 Fax: 029 2043 6801 www.mym.co.uk
Multiple Births Foundation (MBF)	Du Cane Road, London, W12 0HS Tel: 020 8383 3519 Tel: 020 8383 3041 www.multiplebirths.org.uk
National Association for Gifted Children (NAGC)	Elder House, Elder Gate, Milton Keynes, MK9 1LR Tel: 01908 673 677 Fax: 01908 673 679 www.nagcbritain.org.uk
National Association for Special Educational Needs (NASEN)	NASEN House, 4/5 Amber Business Village, Amber Close, Amington, Tamworth, Staffordshire, B77 4RP Tel: 01827 311 500 Fax: 01827 313 005 www.nasen.org.uk
National Association of Toy and Leisure Libraries (Play Matters)	68 Churchway, London, NW1 1LT Tel: 020 7387 9592 Fax: 020 7383 2714 www.charitynet.org/~NATLL
National Autistic Society (NAS)	393 City Road, London, EC1V 1NG Tel: 020 7833 2299 Fax: 020 7833 9666 www.oneworld.org/autism_uk
National Childbirth Trust (NCT)	Alexandra House, Oldham Terrace, London, W3 6NH Tel: 020 8992 8637 Fax: 020 8992 5929 www.nct-online.org
National Childminding Association (NCMA)	8 Masons Hill, Bromley, Kent, BR2 9EY Tel: 020 8464 6164 Fax: 020 8290 6834 www.ncma.org.uk

National Children's Bureau	8 Wakely Street, London, EC1V 7QE Tel: 020 7843 6000 Fax: 020 7278 9512 www.ncb.org.uk
National Council for One Parent Families (NCOPF)	255 Kentish Town Road, London, NW5 2LX Tel: 0800 018 5026 Fax: 020 7482 4851 www.oneparentfamilies.org.uk
National Deaf Children's Society (NDCS)	15 Dufferin Street, London, EC1Y 8UR Tel: 020 7250 0123 Fax: 020 7251 5020 www.ndcs.org.uk
National Early Years Network	77 Holloway Road, London, N7 8JZ Tel: 020 7607 9573 Fax: 020 7700 1105
National Eczema Society (NES)	163 Eversholt Street, London, NW1 1BU Tel: 020 7388 4097 Fax: 020 7388 5882 www.eczema.org
National Library for the Handicapped Child	Try calling 0845 604 0414 on Monday
The National Meningitis Trust	Fern House, Bath Road, Stroud, Gloucestershire, GL5 3TJ Tel: 01453 768000 Fax: 01453 768001 www.meningitis-trust.org.uk Helpline: 0845 6000 800
National Newpin	Sutherland House, 35 Sutherland Square, London, SE17 3EE Tel: 020 7703 6326 Fax: 020 7701 2660
National Playbus Association (NPA)	93 Whitby Road, Brislington, Bristol, BS4 3QF Tel: 0117 911 5375 Fax: 0117 972 1838 playbus@playbus.org.uk
National Portage Association (NPA)	127 Monks Dale, Yeovil, Somerset BA21 3JE Tel: 01935 471641
National Society for the Prevention of Cruelty to Children (NSPCC)	NSPCC National Centre, 42 Curtain Road, London, EC2A 3NH Tel: 020 7825 2500 Fax: 020 7825 2525 www.nspec.org.uk
NCH Action for Children	85 Highbury Park, London, N5 1UD Tel: 020 7226 2033 Fax: 020 7226 2537 www.nchasc.org.uk

Northern Ireland Preschool Playgroups Association (NIPPA)	6C Wildflower Way, Apollo Road, Belfast, BT12 6TA Tel: 02890 662 825 Fax: 02890 381 270 www.nippa.org
One Parent Families Scotland	13 Gayfield Square, Edinburgh EH1 3NX Tel: 0131 556 3899/4563 Fax: 0131 557 9650 www.gn.apc.org/opfs
Parent Network	44–46 Caversham Road, London NW5 2DS Tel: 020 7485 8535 Fax: 020 7267 4426
Parenting Education and Support Forum	Unit 431, Highgate Studios, 53–79 Highgate Road, London NW5 1TL Tel: 020 7284 8370 Fax: 020 7485 3587 www.pesf@dial.pipex.com
Parentline Plus	Unit 520 Highgate Studios, 53–57 Highgate Road, London NW5 1TL Tel: 020 7284 5500 Fax: 020 7284 5501 www.parentlineplus.org.uk
Playgroup Network	PO Box 84, Middlesborough T57 0XT Tel: 0191 230 5520
Pre-School Learning Alliance	69 Kings Cross Road, London WC1X 9LL Tel: 020 7833 0991 Fax: 020 7837 4942 www.pre-school.org.uk
Qualifications and Curriculum Authority (QCA)	83 Picadilly, London, W10 8QA Tel: 020 7509 5555 Fax: 020 7509 6666 www.qca.org.uk
Race Equality Unit (REU)	Unit27/28 Angel Gate, London EC1V 2PT Tel: 020 7278 2331 Fax: 020 7278 8808 www.reunet.demon.co.uk
Reach – The National Advise Centre for Children with Reading Difficulties	California Country Park, 9 Mile End, Finch Hampstead, Berkshire RG40 4HT Tel: 0118 973 7575
Refugee Council	3 Bondway, London SW8 1SJ Tel: 020 7820 3000 Fax: 020 7582 9929
Royal National Institute for the Blind (RNIB)	224 Great Portland Street, London W1N 6AA Tel: 020 7388 1266 Fax: 020 7388 2034 www.rnib.org.uk

Royal Society of Mental Handicapped Children and Adults (MENCAP)	Mencap National Centre, 123 Golden Lane, London EC1Y 0RT Tel: 020 7454 0454 Fax: 020 608 3254 www.mencap.org.uk
Royal Society for the Prevention of Accidents (RoSPA)	Edgbaston Park, 353 Bristol Road, Birmingham B5 7ST Tel: 0121 248 2000 Fax: 0121 248 2001 www.rospa.org.uk
Save the Children (SCF)	17 Grove Lane, London SE5 8RD Tel: 020 7703 5400 Fax: 020 7703 2278 www.savethechildren.org.uk
Scope	6 Market Road, London N7 9PW Tel: 020 7619 7100 Fax: 020 7619 7399 www.scope.org.uk
Scottish Childminding Association (SCMA)	Suite 3, 7 Melville Terrace, Stirling FK8 2ND Tel: 01786 445377 Fax: 01786 449062 www.dialspace.dial.pipex.com\childminding
Scottish Pre-School Play Association (SPPA)	SPPA Centre, 14 Elliot Place, Glasgow G3 8EP Tel: 0141 221 4148 Fax: 0141 221 6043
Sense, The National Deafblind and Rubella Association	11–13 Clifton Terrace, Finsbury Park, London N4 3SR Tel: 020 7272 7774 Fax: 020 7272 6012 Minicom: 020 7272 9648 www.sense.org.uk
Shelter	88 Old Street, London EC1V 9HU Tel: 020 7505 2000 Fax: 020 7505 2169 www.shelter.org.uk
Sickle Cell Society	54 Station Road, Harlesden, London NW10 4UA Tel: 020 8961 7795 Fax: 020 8961 8346 www.sicklecellsociety.org.uk
Soldiers' Sailors' and Airmen's Families Association (SSAFA)	SSAFA Central Office, 19 Queen Elizabeth Street, London SE1 2LP Tel: 020 7403 8783 Fax: 020 7403 8815 www.ssafa.org.uk
Stillbirth and Neonatal Death Society (SANDS)	28 Portland Place, London W1N 4DE Tel: 020 7436 7940 Fax: 020 7436 3715 www.uk-sands.org.uk

Twins and Multiple Births Association (TAMBA)

Harnott House, 309 Charter Road, Little Sutton, Ellesmere Port CH66 1QQ
Tel: 0151 348 0020   Fax: 0870 121 4001   www.tamba.org.uk

Wales Pre-School Playgroups Associations (Wales PPA)

Ladywell House, Newton, Powys, SY16 1JB
Tel: 01686 624573   Fax: 01686 624577   www.walesppa.org.uk

Working Group Against Racism in Children's Resources (WGARCR)

Lady Margaret Hall, 460 Wandsworth Road, London SW8 3LX
Tel: 020 627 4594   Fax: 020 7622 9208

Index

Page numbers in **bold** type refer to illustrations and tables